SUPERCHARGE
YOUR
GUT

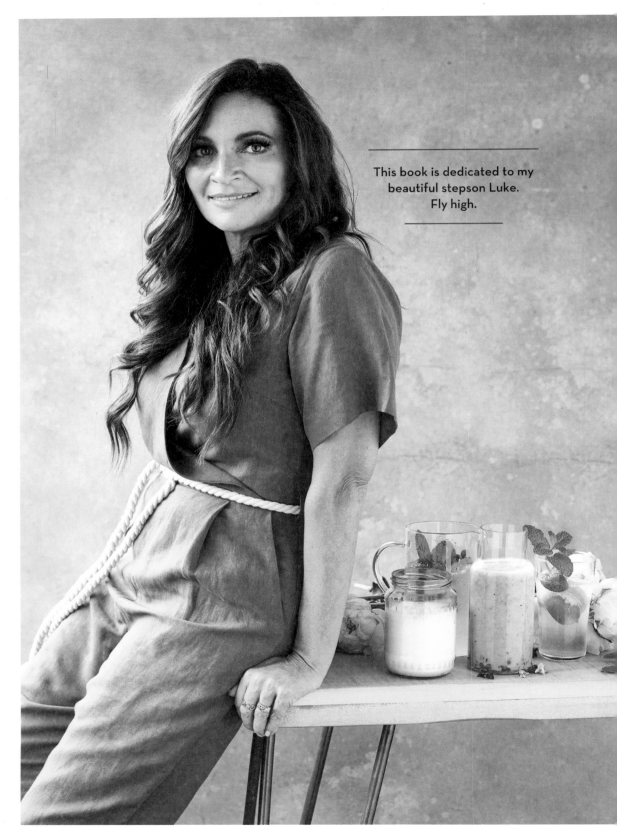

This book is dedicated to my
beautiful stepson Luke.
Fly high.

SUPERCHARGE
YOUR
GUT

LEE HOLMES

MURDOCH BOOKS
SYDNEY · LONDON

FOREWORD

Everything starts in your gut. I've learned that first-hand, witnessed it repeatedly among my patients, and research confirms it: gut health affects how your body feels, how well your mind performs, and... well, *everything*. Whether you want to lose weight, have more energy, prevent disease, or all of the above — mind your gut. It's that simple.

As a medical doctor who specialises in gut health, I've seen how an out-of-whack gut can create immense suffering. I've also seen how a healthy gut can be the key to incredible wellness.

Happiness literally begins in your gut, which manufactures about 95 per cent of your feel-good neurotransmitter, serotonin. An unhealthy gut means you're not producing sufficient amounts of serotonin and about 30 other neurotransmitters, spelling trouble for your mental health and happiness.

Fixing gut imbalances can also help resolve pain, inflammation, fatigue, allergies, asthma and autoimmune diseases, all while helping you get lean and full of energy.

Simply put, health or disease begins in your gut.

That's the underlying premise of Lee Holmes' amazing *Supercharge Your Gut*. Want the next-best prescription to a visit at my clinic to fix your gut? Read this book. Within these pages is everything you need to know to begin your gut-healing journey.

As Lee's story vividly demonstrates, gut imbalances can impact nearly every aspect of your body. I consistently see this in my own practice: headaches, migraines, allergies, autoimmunity, weight gain, acne, skin rashes, yeast infections, hormonal imbalances, fatigue, immune challenges, even the way you sense pain — they all relate to the condition and health of your gut.

Everything you are exposed to — from the antibiotics your doctor prescribes, to the pesticides in your food, the toxins in our environment, and even our chemically laden tap water — creates the perfect storm to trigger daily warfare within your gut.

Take our heavily processed diet, full of sugar, processed foods and additives, that allows harmful bacteria and yeast to proliferate. These unfavourable foods turn on genes harmful to your wellbeing. They create problems like leaky gut that trigger inflammation and inhibit nutrient absorption. And they can make an otherwise-healthy gut go downhill very fast.

Your gut microbiome — that diverse ecosystem living inside you, comprising trillions of symbiotic bacteria that help maintain a healthy digestive system — changes and responds to your diet, good or bad. In other words, what you eat moulds the type of microbiome in your gut.

Many patients also struggle with chronic stress, which research shows can challenge healthy gut bacteria and ramp up bad gut bugs. When super-stressed-out patients with gut issues come to see me, they often neglect ('I don't have time!') or dismiss the value of simple self-care strategies such as deep breathing, meditation and yoga.

Here's the good news: whatever your current stage of health, you're not hopeless. You can take control of your gut and start feeling better today with this book.

Diving into a wide array of health concerns, Lee provides clear, easy-to-apply, hands-on strategies to fix these issues by fixing your gut — while also encouraging you to listen to your body and stay connected to the greater whole of yourself, and embracing lifestyle habits such as gentle exercise, stress management, mindfulness, sleep and nutrient intake, which are all important for healing your gut and overall health.

A refreshing remedy to our fast-paced, ultra-hectic modern diet and lifestyle, *Supercharge Your Gut* is the ultimate how-to manual for fixing your gut, providing troubleshooting advice, along with foods to eat and avoid on this healing journey. To get started, you'll find a day-by-day personal plan that helps you put everything into action.

Oh, and those recipes... If you think healing your gut means deprivation or some bland, boring meal plan, you're going to be surprised with dishes like Chocolate Chilli Beef, Bananacado Bread and even a decadent hot chocolate! And the Mocha & Banana Smoothie Bowl might become your new favourite reason to get up early — who needs stale muffins and sugary lattes? You'll also find delicious nut milks, gut-healing broths, soups and sides that will appeal to vegetarians and meat-eaters equally, while satisfying your family and helping everyone restore and maintain their gut health.

This inspiring, insightful, beautifully presented book provides all the knowledge and guidance you need to fix your gut and create the vibrant health you deserve.

Here's to your *happy gut* — and your *happy life*!

Dr Vincent Pedre M.D.
Functional Medicine Certified Physician
Author of *Happy Gut: The Cleansing Program To Help You Lose Weight, Gain Energy, and Eliminate Pain*

CONTENTS

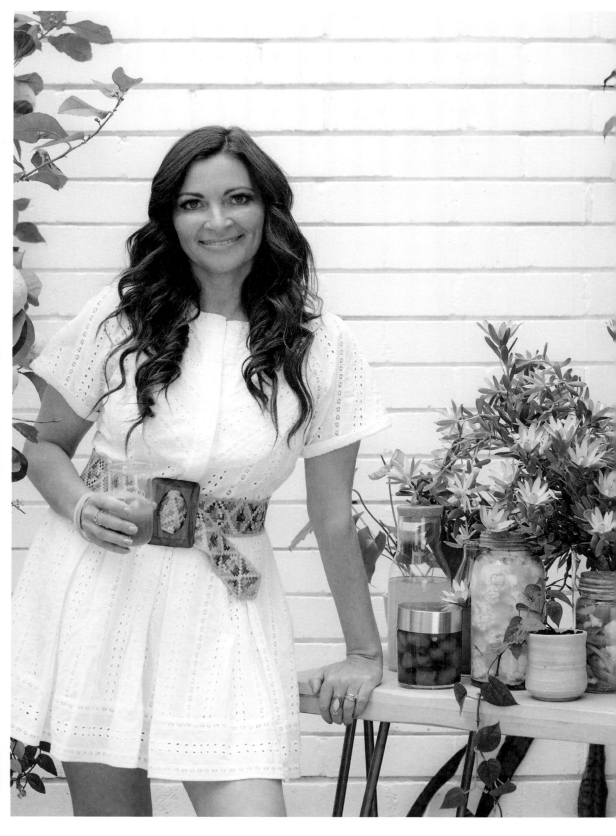

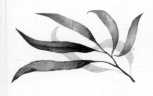

ABOUT ME

Hello. I'm Lee and I'm a food and nutrition coach, wholefood chef and yoga teacher. Seven years ago, I enjoyed a fast-paced career with the ABC in Sydney, helping to promote acts like The Wiggles and Bananas in Pyjamas, when I suddenly became ill.

I felt so unwell I could scarcely haul myself out of bed and go to work, but at the time I chalked it up to life without a pause button. I was a busy working single parent and I was used to feeling tired, but somehow this felt different. I didn't realise back then that I would become one of the 1 in 20 people who are diagnosed with autoimmune diseases in Australia — startlingly, most of them women. My body's immune system had somehow gone haywire and turned on itself, covering my entire body with mystery hives and leaving clumps of hair on my pillow.

My gut had always been a weak point for most of my life, but now it was affecting so much more than just my digestion; my symptoms were sudden and pronounced and I hardly recognised myself. I was dealing with some serious brain fog, aches and pains, and chronic fatigue, and my weight quickly plummeted to 42 kilograms. I was just all over the place. Over the next few months, I saw specialist after specialist. Eventually, after lots of eye-rolling, head-nodding and to-ing and fro-ing, I was diagnosed with non-specific autoimmune disease and fibromyalgia.

MY BREAKING POINT

During my time in and out of hospital, I was given truckloads of steroids, antibiotics and immunosuppressant drugs, which only made me feel worse, due to their long list of side effects. Daily, it felt like an uphill battle. I couldn't differentiate between the side effects of the medication and the symptoms of my condition, but I got my doctors onside and they agreed to allow me to wean myself off the medication, if I started to improve with dietary changes.

I began to simplify my diet and lessened the number of triggers (such as food additives, MSG and highly processed foods) that were making my situation worse, and it was then that I noticed a big improvement in my health: my puffiness subsided, my hives disappeared and my energy levels were improving. I learnt how to give my body intuitively what it needed to feel better, and I also discovered something even more key — supporting yourself matters.

To me, one of the most earth-rocking discoveries was the impact that the gut has on the immune system, and the links that were becoming apparent between diet, digestion and improved immunity. At a young age I had been placed on six consecutive rounds of antibiotics for chronic interstitial cystitis, and not realising how this would affect my gut microbiome I continued taking them, one course after another. This was the beginning of my decline in health, but it wasn't until I was in my 40s that the majority of my problems started.

With my newfound energy and interest in establishing links between my diet and the symptoms I was experiencing, I researched the medicinal capabilities of ingredients and how they could be used to improve my health. I started creating recipes in my kitchen, and from there planted seeds that became the roots of my blog, **superchargedfood.com**. I began to document my process, discoveries and easy-to-concoct — not to mention *digest* — recipes, in the hope of helping people who were suffering similar health experiences. Through my blog, I found a large community of others to share and compare notes with. My way of communicating was through food, a sympathetic ear and a sense of understanding.

I've gone on to publish seven best-selling books featuring easy, nutritious recipes that not only taste delicious and are simple to make, but also help to make you feel amazing. My desire was, and still is, to make healthy eating delicious and simple for everyone, and my area of special interest is the gut.

Do you have a lot going on? Same. I do realise life is busy and that you probably have a lot on your plate. Let me help by making that plate a little more healing for you.

When it comes to gut health, you get out what you put in!

SUPERCHARGE YOUR GUT

Imagine what it would be like to really pay attention to your gut. Have you ever thought about it? There must be a reason you have this book in your hands right now, and I'm excited that you do.

Maybe you've picked up this book because you want to learn more about your gut and the way it influences your health — or perhaps you're suffering from a health issue that is aggravated by diet and a poorly functioning digestive system. It could be an autoimmune or digestive disorder, food allergies or intolerances, inflammatory bowel disease or irritable bowel syndrome, Crohn's disease, coeliac disease, leaky gut, inflammatory issues, thyroid problems, neurological disorders, obesity, diabetes, arthritis or fibromyalgia.

I know that this book came into your hands for a reason, and I'm really glad that it did, because the moment you chose this book, your internal healing began. Think of it as a tool for recovery, and a pathway to freedom from pain, fatigue and digestive distress. I invite you to dive into *Supercharge Your Gut* with open arms, as I gently guide you to an improved way of eating and a new awareness of what it feels like to be energised and supported.

Gut health is becoming one of the most researched topics in the medical realm, and for good reason. The cells in our microbiome at times outnumber our own cells, and we're just beginning to recognise how huge an impact our inner bacteria have on the health of our immune system, our skin, our weight, and even our mental health.

The vital importance of gut health has been understood for thousands of years, with Hippocrates, the father of modern medicine, asserting that 'All disease begins in the gut'. However, it seems that this wisdom has slipped through our fingers. In fact, much of our modern lifestyle is an assault on our gut health — chlorine and fluoride within our water supply, hormones and chemicals in our animal products, caesarean births, formula feeding, processed foods, pesticides, stress, and our Western war on germs (with the overuse of antibacterial cleaning products and antibiotics) all playing a part in throwing our body's microbiome off balance.

An unbalanced inner ecosystem, also known as dysbiosis, can set us up for a range of health problems and illnesses including brain fog, mental health issues, weight gain, diabetes, allergies and autoimmune conditions.

The six rounds of broad-spectrum antibiotics that I took upset my bacterial balance, disturbing my inner ecology. Back then, I didn't have the knowledge or the tools to reset and restore that balance. This is what eventually left my system open to attack, and I believe led to the development of my autoimmune issues.

Our microbiome's genes can vary vastly from person to person, which explains why some people can seemingly eat whatever they like without weight gain or health problems, while others maintain a strict and squeaky-clean diet and suffer from a range of digestive issues and chronic conditions.

The good news is that you have the power to change your gut microbiome and improve your health. The average lifespan of a bacterium within your gut microbiome is 20 minutes! That's the time it takes to drink a cup of coffee, or dandelion tea in my case. This means there's hope throughout your day to make positive choices that will influence the population of your gut microbes towards an inner ecology that will improve your mental and emotional health, increase your energy, boost your immune system and set you up for greater wellness.

My previous book *Heal Your Gut* and the accompanying four-week online program were created to offer you all the tools and recipes to improve your gut health. Hopefully, by incorporating that protocol into your daily life, you have now moved from a place of simply tolerating your gut and those annoying symptoms you thought were a normal part of life, into a new relationship with it.

Loving your gut means understanding its needs and the way it ticks, applying that knowledge through improved daily habits and delicious gut-friendly recipes, and watching as that bloating and digestive pain that you thought were normal begin to disappear.

By reading this book, you'll learn to form an empathetic and nurturing relationship with your gut, where you shift from disassociation towards listening to your gut and what it's telling you, to developing a relationship of gratitude with this wonderful part of your body. The brain fog will lift, your energy will increase, and you'll gain a new sense of vitality that will make way for you to thrive in life, rather than simply survive.

Perhaps you've already read or participated in the *Heal Your Gut* approach and would like to carry on with maintaining your thriving gut by applying gut-healthy principles a couple of days per week. Or perhaps you're new to gut health and want to take a slow and measured approach.

For whatever reason you're here, the gut maintenance plan outlined in this book is a really simple routine you can incorporate into your weekly rhythm, which can act as a short 'rest and digest' break within your week. And the good news is you only need to do it twice a week to see results.

It offers the perfect opportunity for self-care within a busy lifestyle. Everyone needs time within their week to slow down and to really nurture and nourish themselves. This is even more vital if you're a parent or in full-time work or study, where it can be so easy to focus outside yourself for long periods of time.

The convenience options that come with a full life will often place the greatest burden on your gut — takeaway and additive-laden fast foods, mindless snacking or forgetting to eat — robbing your body of important nutrients.

The rush of life can detract from personal self-care, but your gut really needs you to give it some love, and that's why this book has ended up in your helping hands.

Just a couple of days a week, I'd love you to try the recipes and follow the advice from this book, and see the lift in energy and immunity they bring you. You *will* notice the difference, and you *can* learn to not only care for your gut, but also supercharge it for life, with positive consequences for your health and wellbeing.

Enjoy the adventure as you learn how to nurture your gut and find your own way to health and wellness.

Lee xo

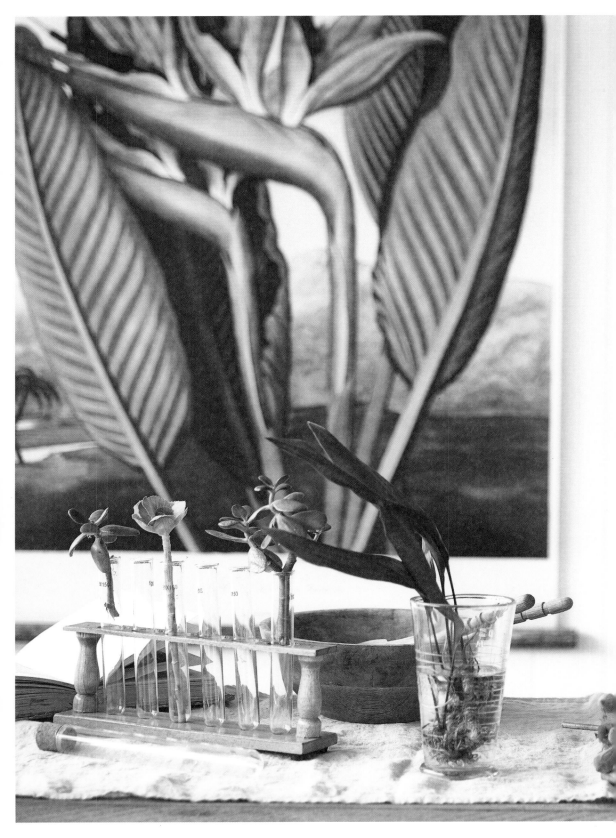

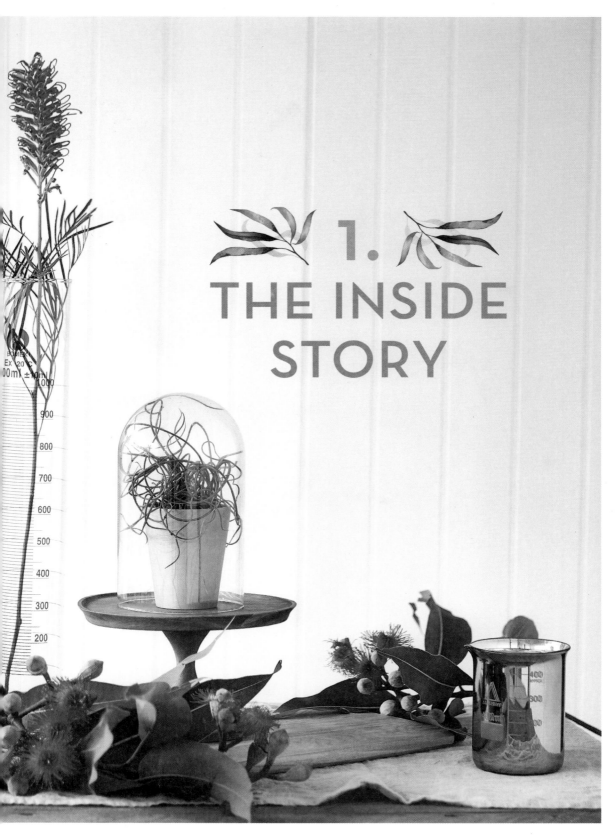

1.
THE INSIDE STORY

THE SECRET LIFE OF THE GUT

If you've been on the journey with me in discovering the amazing world of healing the gut, you'd be well aware that this important part of our anatomy holds colossal value for our overall health. The gut has a secret life of its own that scientists are learning more about every day.

Much more is becoming known about the relationship between our microbiome and our immune system, as well as how the health of our gut and the communication between our microbes and our brain, through the vagus nerve, can have an enormous impact on our mental health and mood.

These are huge findings, but the beauty of the gut is that there is much more to uncover, and layer upon layer of new ways to understand how the gut affects many more aspects of our body.

If we want to optimise our health, we need to start from within. When I talk about the gut I'm talking about *all* of it, from the tongue to the tooshie; I'm not just referring to the tube our food travels through. In this book I'm covering its many layers — the walls of the gut, its living ecosystem or microbiome and the bacteria that comprise it, and also the immune and nervous systems in and around its boundaries.

The gut flora, or gut bacteria, that reside within you play a paramount role in your nutrition and the functioning of your immune system. With the surging use of antibiotics in the post–World War II 'chemical revolution' era, and increasing consumption of mass-produced refined food products and sugars, our microbiomes have become compromised. It's not surprising that there has been a significant rise in allergies and other immune-related conditions in children and adults in recent decades.

Did you know that a massive 80 per cent of your immune system is located within the walls of your intestines? It requires a healthy balance of probiotic (good) bacteria to produce B vitamins for energy, as well as folic acid and vitamin K, which are highly important during pregnancy for foetal development and infant health.

The inner surface area of your small intestine is greater than that of a tennis court.

Probiotic bacteria and a strong intestinal wall structure can also reduce the incidence of food allergies. When the gut barrier is weak and permeable, your immune defences are impaired, and when the number of pathogenic (bad) bacteria is out of control, they can emit toxic substances that can freely enter your bloodstream, which can create problems with autoimmunity and allergies.

A healthy balance of gut flora is important for the production of enzymes and proteins that defend against harmful bacteria. It also stimulates the healthy generation of immunoglobulin A, an antibody that fights infection. The gut microbiome, through its complex interaction with our foods, can have a big impact on nutrient balance, obesity and insulin resistance. A healthy microbiome regulates your metabolism to help you avoid weight gain, by preventing the growth of pathogenic bacterial strains, which increase the body's retention of calories. Studies have shown that when an unhealthy obese mouse microbiome (lower in diversity and good bacteria) is planted into a healthy mouse, the healthy mouse becomes obese too.[1] Therefore, maintaining healthy bacterial colonies (general gut health) is something to consider for weight management.

Balanced gut flora also support positive mood and emotional wellbeing. Evidence shows that psychological distress can be significantly improved when certain probiotic bacteria are present. More about that later.

Another interesting way your gut affects your body is the hold that it has over your energy levels. You might blame your busy lifestyle, but in actual fact it could be your gut that's holding you back — your microbiome plays an important role in the harvest, storage and expenditure of energy obtained from the food you eat. Who knew?

The genome of your gut microbiome actually has a larger coding capacity than the human genome, which means that it also has an additional metabolic capacity, which affects your ability to obtain energy from your diet — impacting fat and sugar metabolism.

The microbes in your gut will convert carbohydrates, proteins and fats in your colon into short-chain fatty acids through fermentation, which are then absorbed and converted into energy, and transported to various tissues and organs around your body.

For example, acetic acid is a short-chain fatty acid produced in the colon that enters your bloodstream to be metabolised by tissues and organs such as the liver, where it is used for fat and cholesterol synthesis. Specific short-chain fatty acids may even reduce the risk of developing a range of gut disorders and cardiovascular disease.[2] Short-chain fatty acids absorbed in the colon are estimated to account for 6–10 per cent of our entire energy production, and the way you can increase this in your own body is to eat more dietary fibre.[3] A daily intake of fibre-rich fruits and vegetables can have a significant impact on energy balance due to the other roles that these fibres play in interaction with your gut microbiome.

Our microbiome is made up of bacteria and other microbes, such as fungi. The microbial genes they carry are responsible for metabolising carbohydrate (starches, sucrose, glucose, galactose and other sugars),[4] affect our absorption of nutrients, and also stimulate lipogenesis (the metabolic formation of fat).

Not only that, your gut is the home of your hydration. Every day as you drink water, it enters the large intestine, where approximately 80 per cent of it is absorbed. The movement of water across your cell membranes occurs by osmosis in the small intestine, where there is a tight coupling between the absorption of water and dissolved nutrients. Hydration is very important for the functioning of your entire body, but it all starts in the gut.

Drinking plenty of water keeps your intestines smooth and flexible. A hydrated gut also helps keep food moving through your intestines, and ultimately allows food waste to exit your body, which is also important for detoxification. One of the main causes of chronic constipation is dehydration — if your body doesn't have enough water, your stools will become hard and difficult to pass, leading to a build-up of toxins on the intestinal wall, which, combined with leaky gut, can be problematic. To keep hydrated, women need an average daily water intake of around 2.2 litres (75 fl oz), and men 3 litres (100 fl oz).[5]

These are just a few of the scientific connections that have been made between the health of the gut and our overall health, with more links being made as researchers consider the vast ripple effect that this invisible community has on all of our body's functions.

What is becoming increasingly clear is that this living, mysterious life force within us will do our health a whole lot of good if we take the time to nurture it and treat it with the best of care.

THE AGES AND STAGES OF GUT HEALTH

To give your gut the real support it needs, it's helpful to understand how a healthy gut microbiome is formed.

Before birth, we're all more or less sterile — we have no microbes. Within a few years, we're covered in thousands of different species of microbes colonising every millimetre of our body that is exposed to the outside world. By the time we start school, we have vastly different populations living in the different habitats around our bodies. Even as adults and into old age, our microbiota continues to shift.

BIRTH AND INFANCY

Within the womb, you were living in the sterile environment of amniotic fluid. In a vaginal birth, a baby's nasal passages, eyes and skin are colonised with the mother's bacteria, forming the beginning of the baby's immune system. When a newborn begins to feed from the breast, the unique oligosaccharides contained in this miraculous milk pass through the baby's small intestine unharmed, landing in the large intestine, where they literally feed the initial seeding of the mother's bacteria imparted during birth, initiating the wonderful beginning of the child's microbiome.

CHILDHOOD

Microbial populations shift and change a lot during early childhood. There's also much variation among individuals, depending upon whether they've been breast or formula fed, the diet they're introduced to, and if they've been given antibiotics as a result of the array of childhood illnesses that come in the early years of life. For all these reasons, variation of microbes in the gut is highest during childhood.

There's growing recognition that the microbiome is directly linked to infant and childhood development and immunity. For example, it's now known that the use of antibiotics, especially in the first 12 months of life, creates significant decreases in the number of *Bifidobacterium* and *Bacteroides*, and a reduced bacterial diversity, which is important for a robust immune system. Avoiding antibiotics where possible, replenishing and supporting diversity through child-appropriate probiotics and having a good diet with fermented foods is important for building a strong gut and immune system into the further stages of life.

ADOLESCENCE

As children grow into teenagers and young adults, they become more independent about their food and lifestyle choices — relying primarily on their amygdala (the emotional, impulsive part of the brain) before their brain reaches full maturity in their mid-20s. Teens and adolescents may choose unhealthy processed and sugar-laden foods, or experiment with alcohol and drugs, all of which have negative effects on the microbiome.

Eating too many grains, sugars and processed foods serves as a 'feast' for pathogenic microorganisms and yeasts, causing them to multiply rapidly. As the healthy balance of species is altered, this can lead to digestive issues, nutrient deficiencies, lowered immunity and even behavioural and mental health issues, as healthy vagus nerve communication to the brain is compromised. Helping our young people by limiting their access to heavily processed foods, and nourishing them with *real* foods, will go a long way towards nurturing their microbiome, and influencing them to pursue a healthy lifestyle into their future.

THE WORKING YEARS

After a young person leaves home, independence is in full motion. They enter the world of work or study, find employment, perhaps become a spouse, begin a family, encounter mortgage and financial stresses, and experience the busiest season of life.

Stress plays a major role in gut health. It has been shown that different types of psychological stress — including maternal separation, chronic social distress, restraint conditions, crowding, heat stress and acoustic stress — can alter the composition of the gastrointestinal microbiota; and likewise, an unhealthy diversity of bacteria can impact on emotional behaviour and stress response.[6]

If an adult hasn't inherited healthy eating habits from their family or community, chances are that in this time of life, they'll choose the convenience of processed food, which is detrimental for the microbiome. Modern processed foods can be difficult to digest, placing a burden on the gut. 'Leaky gut' is a classic symptom emerging in these years if the gut hasn't been looked after with proper diet and lifestyle; others include autoimmune conditions, new allergies, depression, anxiety and recurrent colds and flus. Estimated to comprise trillions of microbes — together possessing 100 times the number of genes in the human genome — it's no wonder the state of an adult's microbiome can influence so many aspects of their physiology and health.

SENIOR YEARS

The state of our microbiome in the older years may be a big key to how well we age, and our resistance to illness and degenerative disease.

Studies have shown an association between microbial diversity and the functional independence of elderly individuals. Reduced microbial diversity has been correlated with decreased dietary diversity, increased physical frailty, raised levels of inflammatory markers, and the occurrence of cancers and digestive and atherosclerotic diseases. Elderly people living in the community have been found to have the most diverse microbiota, and have more robust health than those in short- or long-term residential care.[7]

Taking special care to nourish or restore the microbiome of older adults holds promise as an innovative strategy that may help slow down the development of illnesses associated with ageing.

THE MULTICULTURAL GUT

I'd like you to think of your gut as if it were like the depths of the Amazonian rainforest. It's a dense, complex ecosystem that requires a balance of diversity in order to sustain its beauty. It's also a large landscape that requires careful curating.

Every unique part of this ecosystem plays a particular microscopic role on its own — but together, the vast array of relationships between these parts creates the magnificent, multifaceted splendour of a large-scale, perfectly functioning, natural system. Diminishing the diversity by leaving out, damaging or creating conditions where particular strains of bacteria cannot survive has a cumulative effect on this ecosystem's potential to thrive and protect you.

It's now recognised that our gut flora has its own language, and bacteria can communicate with each other independently. An example of this is that you may eat a certain food and your gut flora could have a biochemical 'conversation' about it; I find this truly astonishing, and fascinating. This was one of the key discoveries I made when interviewing Dr Emeran Mayer, a world-renowned gastroenterologist and neuroscientist, for my Supercharge Your Gut online summit. He spoke about the biochemical dialogue that occurs between the brain, digestive tract, and the trillions of bacteria residing there.[8]

Another way of picturing your gut is to think of it as a geographical society, full of diverse cultures, and experiencing the tapestry of varied beauty that multiculturalism brings. Just like a multicultural and diverse society, we want our digestive systems to have open borders — celebrating and welcoming different communities and cultures from across the globe, in order to contribute to a more wholesome, progressive and healthy civilisation. No walls, no barriers. Let diversity flourish!

Generally, the digestive tracts of the developed Western world look like barren deserts compared with the lush tropical rainforest found in indigenous people. Interestingly, the Yanomami people who dwell in the Venezuelan rainforest have the widest array of microbial genes yet found in a human gut. For thousands of years, some groups have lived with zero contact with the rest of the world, and are believed to be some of the few remaining communities never to have been exposed to antibiotics, which can decimate our microbial communities.

It's believed that the absence of important bacterial species from our Western microbiome — such as those that metabolise carbohydrates, or others that communicate with our immune system — could explain some of our increasingly common immune-related conditions, such as Crohn's disease, multiple sclerosis and other autoimmune disorders. Perhaps, in our Western lifestyle, we have lost species that help our immune system to function normally?

Taking conscious shifts to imitate our hunter–gatherer brothers and sisters seems to be a commonsense approach to promoting the diversity of our dwindling Western microbiome.

Other factors, besides antibiotics, that dismantle microbial diversity include acid-blocking drugs, stress, modern environmental toxins, chemicals in our water supply, pesticides on our food, using antibacterial soaps and cleansers, and the rising preference for planned caesarean sections, which mean that our future generations are experiencing a loss of microbial biodiversity.

But the good news is that we can help increase our microbial diversity by eating a wholefood, organic, varied and colourful diet that includes a range of fermented foods, and drinking clean filtered water.

The intestinal microflora is a complex, diverse ecosystem, and scientists have identified more than 400 different bacterial species within it.

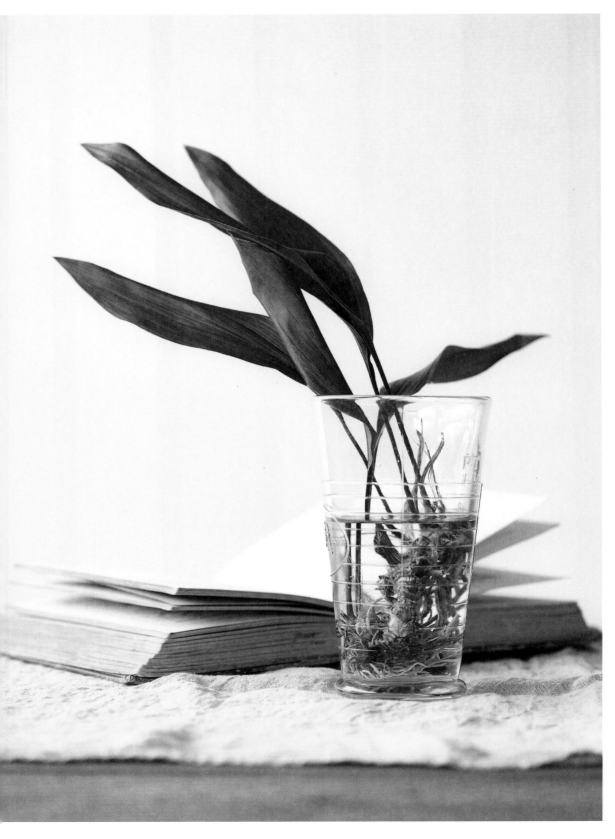

NURTURING THE RAINFOREST WITHIN

Now just for a second, I'd love you to imagine the most exquisite rainforest you've ever seen. Think of every minute detail, from the sound of cute little frogs ribbiting, to the sky-scraping trees watching over, and the beautiful flow of the cleanest streaming rivers. Every small fragment plays a part in a much larger picture. For the rainforest to carry on flourishing, the ecosystem needs to be cared for. The soil needs to be fertile, the plants require watering, and the rivers need rainwater to continue their flow.

Just like the Amazon rainforest, our gut requires the right kind of soil as a foundation for growth. For the trees to germinate, we need to plant and cultivate the appropriate kinds of seeds, and to witness them germinating, maturing and blossoming we need to nourish our inner ecosystem with nutritious and beneficial plant food.

From infancy, the colostrum in breast milk is the 'soil' that helps to nurture our probiotic seeds and develop a healthy microbiota, providing friendly bacteria with a home to grow by keeping any spaces, or leaky junctions, in the gut 'closed'. It also has a huge influence on the composition of our gut, and can reduce the number of pathogens and substances that enter the bloodstream. Without colostrum, the gut's permeability is weakened, which can lead to an inability to absorb essential nutrients.

To create vibrantly coloured plants and shrubbery, we need to introduce a variety of seeds to our soil, in the form of a diverse range of fibre-rich healing foods. To keep our inner woodland flourishing and beautiful, probiotics are also necessary to help the growth of our friendly gut bacteria, which are a large part of our ecosystem. Probiotic-rich foods, such as sauerkraut, kimchi and cultured vegetables, help our inner plants thrive, whereas prebiotics act as a food and fertiliser to help fuel and nourish our probiotics.

Interestingly, the Yanomami people consume a high-fibre diet based largely on cassava (also known as yucca), which contains prebiotic resistant starches that feed diverse communities of good bacteria within the gut. Studies conducted on rats have found that when the animals were deprived of prebiotic fibre, the level of microbial diversity dropped quickly and dramatically. However, once prebiotic fibre was reintroduced into the diet, the level of diversity of the gut organisms significantly improved.

Foods rich in prebiotic fibre include jicama (Mexican yam), onions, garlic, dandelion greens, asparagus, chicory root, cashews, pistachios, lentils, kidney beans and Jerusalem artichoke; more about these later.

Now that we're delving deeper into our exquisite rainforest, remember that, as in any diverse environment, there may be a few nasty little bugs about. The way to combat these is by consuming antifungal and antibacterial foods, such as garlic and coconut oil, which can really help you ward off viruses, bacteria and a variety of infections. You don't want to wipe out all the bad bugs entirely; it's just about having a healthy balance.

Every rainforest adores leafy greens, and so does your inner jungle. Beautiful verdant vegetables and leafy greens have anti-inflammatory properties due to their high vitamin K, vitamin A and vitamin C content, setting strong foundations for a thriving ecosystem.

Want to pretty up your rainforest with daffodils or golden sunflowers? Turmeric is an active anti-inflammatory that will help keep your gut blossoming beautifully.

To keep the rivers flowing and the plants looking fresh, a rainforest needs to be properly hydrated, with clean fresh water. Other wonderful gut-friendly liquids to embrace are herbs and teas, such as ginger, fenugreek, lavender and fennel, which will help you to better assimilate and process the foods you're eating. Keeping hydrated also enables you to balance out the pH of the rainforest, which is necessary for it to flourish and grow. Drinking 30 minutes before (not during) meals can help keep your digestive enzymes firing.

To truly supercharge your gut, you need to ensure you're keeping it clean and tidy. This can be done through intermittent fasting (lowering your daily food intake to 2100 kJ/500 calories for women and 2500 kJ/600 calories for men), and taking cleansing ingredients such as food-grade diatomaceous earth (see page 43). Intermittent fasting with wholefoods enables the digestive system to rest and restore; you can read more in my book *Fast Your Way to Wellness*.

Our inner rainforest should be a place of harmony and tranquillity. Our emotions can trigger negative symptoms in the gut, which radiate throughout the rest of the body. Looking at what we feed our emotions is just as important as what we physically feed our rainforest, which is why keeping stress levels down and practising mindfulness through techniques such as meditation and yoga are so beneficial to our health and vitality.

Speaking of the mind, next I'd love to enlighten you on the connections between our two brains. Literally two.

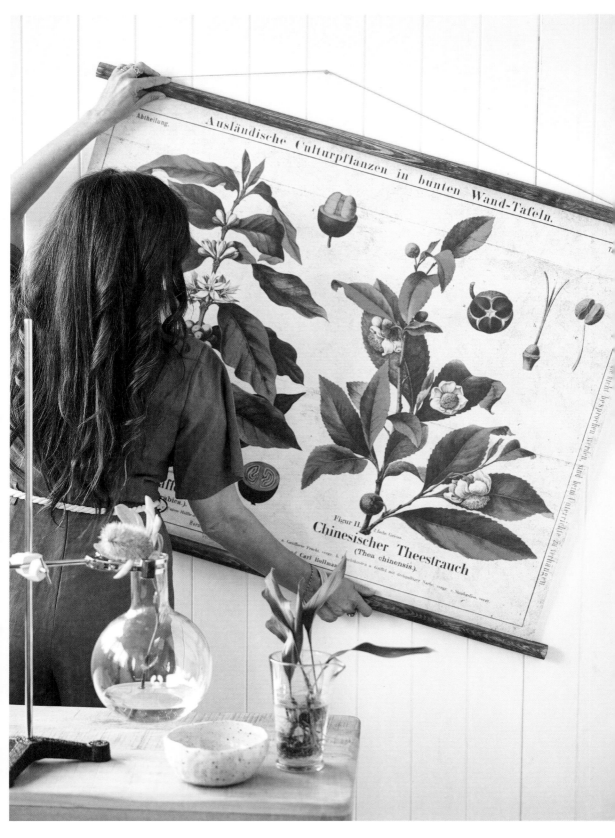

THE CONNECTED GUT

Ever considered what could help drive depression, weight gain, hormonal imbalances, sleepless nights or an attack of the hangries? Read on to discover the complex connections that your gut has influence over, and how they could be affecting you in a myriad of surprising ways.

TWO BRAINS, ONE BODY

This is the tale of two brains. Did you know that not only are our mouth and gut connected, so are our brain and our gut? This is known as the gut–brain axis, and it's so tight-knit and interdependent that it can have a significant impact on mood and behaviour. The gut–brain axis is like an information superhighway that provides constant updates on the state of affairs from your brain to your gut and vice versa.

Ever followed your 'gut feeling' because you actually feel something within your gut telling you which decision to make? Or maybe you've ignored these feelings and found yourself in the wrong place at the wrong time? This isn't just your imagination – you're actually receiving signals from what is known as your 'second brain', which is hidden within the walls of your digestive system, and is linked to a wide range of functions including digestion, mood and overall health.

Although our 'second brain' doesn't make executive decisions like our actual brain, the two do communicate back and forth via electrical impulses through a pathway of nerves – the gut–brain axis – and this pathway influences our endocrine, immune and neural systems.

The second brain – more scientifically known as the enteric nervous system – is found in your gastrointestinal tract and is made up of two thin layers, comprising more than 100 million nerve cells. Its main role is controlling digestion, including the release of digestive enzymes, nutrient absorption and the elimination of waste. During foetal growth the enteric nervous system develops from the same tissues as the central nervous system, making its structures and chemical responses very similar to those of the brain.

The communication between your second brain and your actual brain happens via the nervous system, hormones and the immune system; even your microbiome can release neurotransmitters that speak to the brain.

Ever had that feeling in your gut when things don't seem quite right? Or that feeling of butterflies when you're a little nervous? This isn't just a 'feeling' – it's your 'second brain' sending you a signal.

So while your gut bacteria have an impact on the brain, the brain also influences your gut microbiome, in a perpetual feedback loop, to influence your perception of the world and your behaviour.

Now think on this: have you ever suffered an attack of the hangries, or a period of food feistiness? Being nutritionally deprived can have a dramatic effect on the brain and our mood, and it turns out there's a scientific explanation for this. Researchers at Melbourne's Monash University believe ghrelin — the hormone associated with appetite, which is produced in the second brain in your gut — is responsible. The receptors for ghrelin in your brain can cause mood changes and anxiety until you eat something.

Researchers who participated in my Supercharge Your Gut online summit indicated that for every one message that the brain sends to the gut, the gut sends back ten messages to the brain. Inflammation, chronic abdominal pain, eating disorders and psychosocial stressors are all associated with disruptions in brain–gut communication.

A perfect example of these disruptions is the effect that stress can have on both the brain and the gut. Scientific evidence shows that stress can destroy the beneficial bacteria found within the gut. One study showed that during an exam week, stool samples taken from university students contained fewer lactobacilli bacteria than during the relatively untroubled first days of the semester.[9] These stress-induced changes to the microbiome then impact the brain due to defensive molecules produced in the gut during stress, disrupting the brain chemistry and making you more vulnerable to anxiety and depression.[10]

When you're feeling stressed or anxious, your body releases peptides (short chains of amino acids) known as corticotrophin-releasing factors, and these can have a strong effect on the gut, resulting in inflammation and increased gut permeability and sensitivity. Chronic exposure to stress can lead to a variety of gastrointestinal diseases, such as gastro-oesophageal reflux disease, peptic ulcer disease, irritable bowel syndrome, inflammatory bowel disease and even food allergies,[11] due to stress slowing down the transit time of food within the small intestine, encouraging overgrowth of bacteria, and compromising the intestinal barrier.[12]

Have you ever felt upset, anxious or stressed about something, and symptoms such as constipation, diarrhoea and bloating have suddenly appeared as well? Researchers are now beginning to discover that it can also work the other way around — that our enteric nervous system can trigger big emotional shifts, and that gut issues may also be causing those emotional feelings.

Studies are also proving that by treating inflammation in the gut, you can keep feelings of anxiety and depression under control, and by controlling these feelings, you can reduce the amount of inflammation and increase the amount of beneficial bacteria found within the gut.[13]

So how can you offer support to both your gut and your brain? By supporting the growth of healthy gut flora, and encouraging diversity within the gastrointestinal tract you can help reduce hypersensitivity and leaky gut permeability, and normalise brain levels of stress hormones. Improving the quality and health of your friendly gut bacteria can also benefit your mental health and overall wellbeing.

Interestingly, around 90 per cent of your serotonin levels are stored in the gut, with only 5–10 per cent stored in the brain. Serotonin is a neurotransmitter that plays a major role in controlling your mood. The right amount of serotonin will have you feeling relaxed and positive, but imbalances in serotonin contribute to feelings associated with depression, and can also affect your appetite, sleep, memory and social behaviour. Skewed serotonin levels can also cause constipation or diarrhoea.

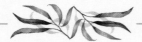

FOODS TO BOOST SEROTONIN — YOUR HAPPY HORMONE!

EGGS can significantly boost your blood plasma levels of tryptophan, the amino acid from which serotonin is biochemically derived.

FOODS HIGH IN VITAMIN B6 such as spinach, cauliflower, garlic, fish, celery, chicken and beef; vitamin B6 plays an important role in helping your body produce serotonin.

FERMENTED FOODS can assist in the digestion and absorption of all the important nutrients you need for serotonin production.

WEIGHT, IS IT MY GUT?

Many of our dietary decisions — whether it's low-fat, low-carb or weight-reducing — are based on how certain foods will affect our physical appearance. Unfortunately, it's usually not until things start to go wrong with our health that we really start to consider what's happening on the inside, in our inner ecosystem. The truth is, what's happening in your gut has a huge impact on how you look, as well as the number that appears on your bathroom scales — and once you realise this, it's easier to make better decisions about food.

Unhealthy diet and not enough exercise are the main causes usually addressed by people battling with weight issues — but now new research is showing that the billions upon billions of bacteria that reside in our gut are playing a major role in both how much we weigh *and* our physical appearance.

This is due to our gut bacteria being able to influence the way we store fat and how our body balances blood glucose levels; these microscopic workers can even alter our feelings of being hungry or full.

When researchers began looking into the role of gut flora in obesity, they discovered that the microbiome within the gut of people at a healthy weight was much more diverse than in those who were overweight. For example, bacteria in the Christensenellaceae family were found in participants with a healthy body mass index, whereas those who were overweight had a lot less of the beneficial bacteria present, if any at all.[14]

One study found that obese women who consumed a probiotic supplement were able to lose twice as much fat over a six-month period as those who did not. The probiotics helped control their appetite, which seemed to decrease as their gut microbiome adapted and became more diverse.[15]

One example of how bacteria can affect your weight involves a microbe known as *Helicobacter pylori*, which is the bacteria that can cause stomach ulcers. Antibiotics have helped manage the detrimental effects of this bacterium, but have also unwittingly contributed to our growing waistlines, because *Helicobacter pylori* also reduces the amount of the hunger hormone ghrelin. When you eat, your ghrelin levels go down, and your appetite goes away. If you don't have *Helicobacter pylori* in your system, your ghrelin levels stay raised, and your brain thinks you still need to eat, resulting in the overconsumption of food.[16]

So, what is the most natural way to support a healthy gut ecosystem? Unsurprisingly, it's my favourite area — food and diet!

There's an abundance of evidence that consuming a diet high in bad fats, refined carbs and low fibre disrupts the balance between good and bad bacteria and favours fat accumulation and obesity. This is why it helps to consume foods that support the growth of beneficial bacteria, which will have you feeling and looking amazing.

HORMONES AND GUT HEALTH

A healthy gut is the tranquil home that brings life to healthy hormones.

Considering the vast influence that hormones have on our health — from controlling blood sugar and weight gain, to menstrual cycles and fertility, the health of our skin, thyroid function and more — the connection between our gut and our hormones is one that can affect us in ways we may not even be aware of.

Gut hormones, which are secreted by cells in the stomach, pancreas and small intestine, influence a range of digestive organs. Studies have shown that most of the gut peptides (short chains of amino acids) act as neurotransmitters and neuromodulators — in other words hormones — in our central and peripheral nervous systems, linking the health of our gut to healthy mood and nervous system functioning.

Gut hormones also play a large role in regulating our weight and appetite. Leptin is the master hormone for regulating our weight, and operates an incredible system in our body that tells us when to eat, when to store fat, and when we need to increase our intake of carbohydrate for energy instead of fat and protein.

The interplay between our communication hormones, such as leptin, involves a complex system of feedback loops that maintain the balance required for our bodies to survive. With the right food and periods of intermittent fasting, this communication and harmony provides us with better health and increased longevity.

For example, enteroglucagon is a peptide hormone located in the small intestine, and has a role in insulin secretion. Cholecystokinin exists in the enteric nerves and is responsible for the feeling of 'fullness' or satiety after a meal, while peptide YY located in the colon inhibits food intake by reducing your appetite. If your gut is in an unhealthy or unbalanced state, can you see how this could be a problem?

With so many hormones controlling our ability to feel satisfied by our food and regulating our blood sugar and appetite, the maintenance of a healthy weight may be greatly helped by the proper care and nourishment of our gut.

Due to our high-carbohydrate and overly processed diets, and our constant need to snack or eat every few hours, many of our gut hormones — especially our master communication hormones such as leptin and insulin — have become overloaded and resistant. They can't register or decipher the messages being communicated to them, which is subsequently having a negative effect on our health, especially when it comes to our appetite and weight.

One of the simple ways to support gut hormones is to avoid a highly processed diet with an excess of sugar and refined carbohydrates.

Following the Supercharge Your Gut principles in this book will help you to shift any excess weight inhibiting the healthy communication between your gut hormones, and change the functioning of your entire body into one that is constructive and health-promoting. Hallelujah to that.

THYROID AND DIGESTIVE HEALTH

Both the thyroid and the gut play a huge role in keeping us functioning properly, but there's also an intimate connection between the two. Poor gut health can suppress thyroid function, and low thyroid function can lead to an inflamed leaky gut.

The thyroid is a butterfly-shaped gland in your neck that produces two types of hormones: thyroxine (T4), which is the inactive thyroid hormone, and triiodothyronine (T3) the active form. Both of these hormones are necessary for all the cells in your body to function properly.

For our thyroid hormones to do their job, T4 needs to be converted into the active T3 form, and 20 per cent of this conversion happens within the gut flora of the large intestine. The conversion can be enhanced by an enzyme called intestinal sulfatase, which is produced by the good bacteria within the gut — so any imbalances in the gut microflora can significantly reduce the conversion.

A major side effect of a gut microbial imbalance is that it impairs gut motility, resulting in constipation. Constipation can decrease the clearance of oestrogen and increase thyroid-binding globulin, a protein that binds to T3, making it chemically inactive and reducing the amount of active thyroid hormone being released into the bloodstream. Inflammation in the gut also reduces active T3 due to raised cortisol levels; cortisol decreases active T3 levels by inhibiting the conversion of T4 to T3.

WAYS TO SUPPORT YOUR THYROID

The good news is you can help support your thyroid hormones by enjoying a gut-healthy diet.

Turmeric can help reduce inflammation and is a delicious addition to your meals; my Turmeric Fudge on page 279 contains this golden ingredient. Plus it's yum times five!

My delicious Maca & Tahini Latte on page 139 can help support the immune system and improve the circulation of hormones. Maca stimulates and nourishes the hypothalamus and pituitary glands, which are the 'master glands' of the body. These glands actually regulate the other glands, so when in balance they can bring harmony to the adrenal, thyroid, pancreas, ovarian and testicular glands[17] — which is wonderful if, like me, you're in your 50s and in the menopausal stage of life.

Bone broths (pages 192–198) are another magical meal that supports thyroid function. Containing zinc, an essential mineral that supports immune function and promotes healing within the gut, as well as iron, bone broths can be added to soups and slow-cooked meals to enhance their flavour and boost gut health.

Invest in iodine-rich foods such as seaweed, seafood and, in smaller amounts, eggs. Eat three Brazil nuts a day to keep selenium levels stable, and say goodbye to gluten.

Having low thyroid hormone levels can also make it difficult for the gut to heal. An inflamed and leaky gut can be supported by the methods on the following page.

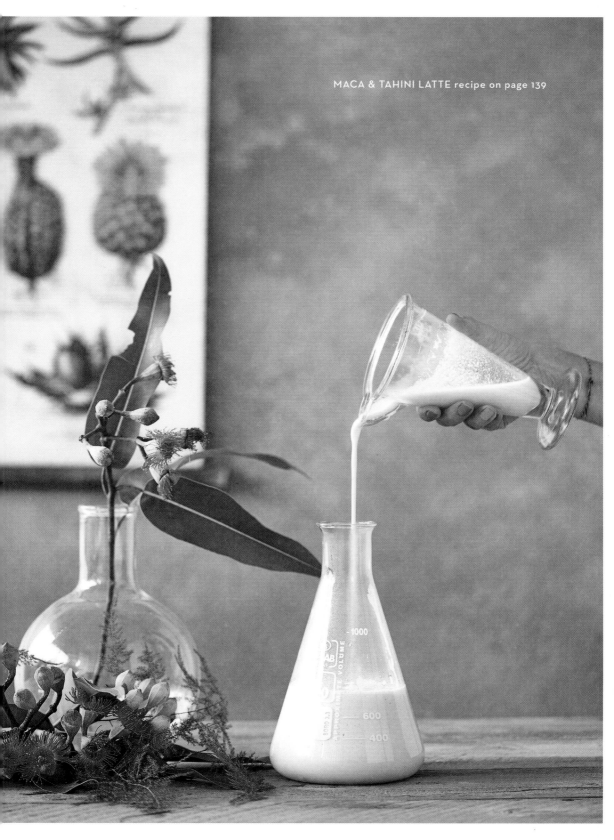

MACA & TAHINI LATTE recipe on page 139

REMOVING LEAKY GUT TRIGGERS

These include foods such as gluten, sugar and dairy products, which can all cause damage to your intestinal lining and contribute to leaky gut — where the intestinal wall becomes permeable to proteins, which then make their way into the bloodstream. This can cause abnormal immune responses, allergies, intolerances and autoimmune diseases.

REDUCING STRESS

Stress will weaken your immune system and impair your body's ability to fight off foreign invaders such as bad bacteria and viruses, leading to inflammation in the gut, and reducing the amount of inactive thyroid hormone being converted to active thyroid hormone.

EATING FOODS THAT REDUCE INFLAMMATION

Spices, especially ginger and turmeric, are fantastic for reducing inflammation within the gut. Studies have shown that people who consumed turmeric were less likely to suffer from goitre and iodine deficiency, both of which are linked to hypothyroidism, a condition where the thyroid produces insufficient amounts of thyroid hormone.

CONSUMING FOODS CONTAINING ZINC AND IRON

Both of these trace minerals are vital for thyroid function and gut health. Zinc plays an essential role in gut health and healing, and supports immune function. Low zinc can cause T3, T4 and thyroid-stimulating hormone levels to become low, while iron is needed to repair thyroid imbalances, and decreased iron levels can reduce thyroid function.

Containing both zinc and iron, bone broths can be used as a base for soup or sipped throughout the day.

By concentrating on restoring the gut, you're supporting your immune system and hormone production, which will draw you so much closer to feeling good again, and unlock the door to better health.

The gut–thyroid connection is just one of the many important links within the body where your gut holds major influence. By nurturing your gut you're supporting these connections and functions, and that's a big bonus.

THE GUT AND SLEEP

Do you struggle with your shut-eye? Scientists are now uncovering the relationship between our microbial ecosystems and sleep. Yes that's right: our sleep quality is also being linked to the health of our gut.

Sleep is vital to our health and daily functioning, as it's the time when we restore energy and repair our cells; our gut could be the key to unlocking great sleep, with research showing how it profoundly impacts a range of psychological functions, from regulating the hormones that control sleep and wakefulness, to shifting our circadian rhythms and altering our sleep–wake cycle.[18]

I've covered how, right now within your body, there's a complex communication interplay between your microbiome and your brain, and how this can be linked with depression, anxiety and emotional stress; clearly these will have an impact on the quality of your sleep.

An unhealthy balance of microflora has also been shown to increase pain perception, and with the connection between pain and poor sleep very clear, a healthy gut can help minimise the experience of pain, therefore promoting a more peaceful sleep.

The times I was suffering a relapse in my fibromyalgia, I noticed that not only was my sleep interrupted, but my gut didn't seem to be functioning well either, and once I addressed my gut, my sleep patterns improved.

Your circadian rhythm is the 24-hour biological system that maintains and balances sleep and wake cycles, and your microbiome also has its own rhythms that are capable of influencing and disrupting one another. Microbes have a mind of their own, including how they affect our sleep.

The intestinal microbiome both produces and releases serotonin and dopamine, which maintain a healthy mood and sleep patterns. As night-time approaches, your levels of serotonin increase and send signals to the brain to start producing melatonin, the hormone that stimulates sleepiness and controls your sleep cycle. This process

The hormones and neurotransmitters that play a vital role in regulating circadian rhythms are also largely controlled by the gut.

is vital if you want to enjoy a good night's sleep.[19] It has also been proven that healthy bacteria can actually produce serotonin by stimulating the intestinal cells, meaning the healthier your gut is, the better you will sleep.[20]

From the opposite direction, a deficiency of melatonin, known as 'the darkness hormone', has been connected with increased intestinal permeability.

Sleep is the ideal time for your body to regrow, repair, recharge and replenish — but for this to happen, you need to go into a 'deep sleep'. It can take up to four hours to get into this deep sleep stage, and only 25 per cent of our sleeping time is spent in this ideal stage of sleep. This is why it's valuable to get at least 8 hours of sleep — to make sure you're spending enough time in a deep sleep.

When it comes to diet and sleep, try to avoid foods that cause irritation within your gut and immune system, causing issues to flare up at night and disrupt your sleep.

Late-night snackers, hold your horses. My advice for better sleep is to try to eat early and avoid any stimulating, caffeinated or inflammatory foods, aiming for easy-to-digest, nutrient-dense dinners. The superbowls, soups and slow-cooked casseroles in this book are great dinner options, and before dinner you can also incorporate a pre-digestive, which you'll find on pages 146–149. Pre-digestives aid digestion as they contain naturally occurring digestive enzymes, meaning that thankfully, much of the hard work is done for you, allowing your body to focus on absorption.

The beauty of nurturing your gut is that once you've given your digestive system a rest by removing inflammatory foods and repairing the gut lining through wholesome broths and gentle easy-to-digest meals, you've created the conditions for a healthy, robust microbiome — and you'll not only experience improved digestion, but the myriad beneficial effects throughout your body, from a boosted immune system to glowing skin, improved mood, and a more restful night's sleep.

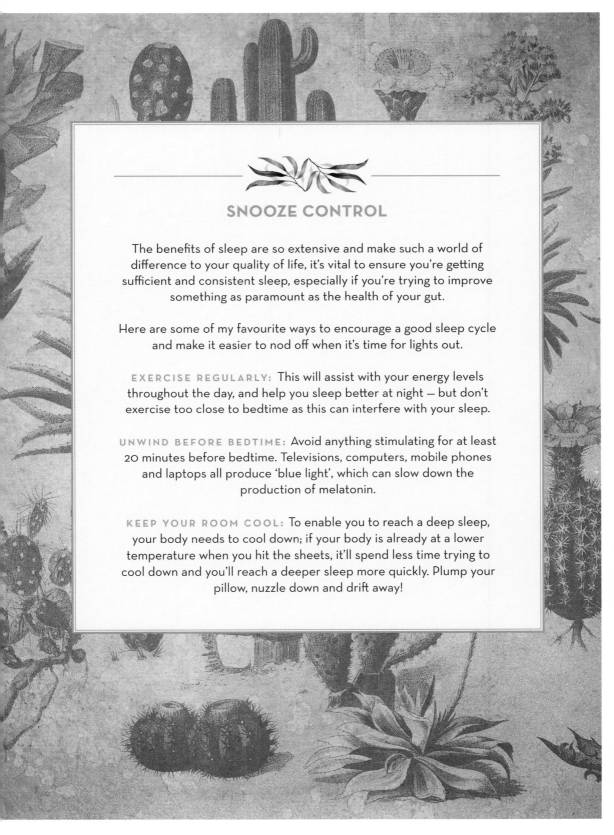

SNOOZE CONTROL

The benefits of sleep are so extensive and make such a world of difference to your quality of life, it's vital to ensure you're getting sufficient and consistent sleep, especially if you're trying to improve something as paramount as the health of your gut.

Here are some of my favourite ways to encourage a good sleep cycle and make it easier to nod off when it's time for lights out.

EXERCISE REGULARLY: This will assist with your energy levels throughout the day, and help you sleep better at night — but don't exercise too close to bedtime as this can interfere with your sleep.

UNWIND BEFORE BEDTIME: Avoid anything stimulating for at least 20 minutes before bedtime. Televisions, computers, mobile phones and laptops all produce 'blue light', which can slow down the production of melatonin.

KEEP YOUR ROOM COOL: To enable you to reach a deep sleep, your body needs to cool down; if your body is already at a lower temperature when you hit the sheets, it'll spend less time trying to cool down and you'll reach a deeper sleep more quickly. Plump your pillow, nuzzle down and drift away!

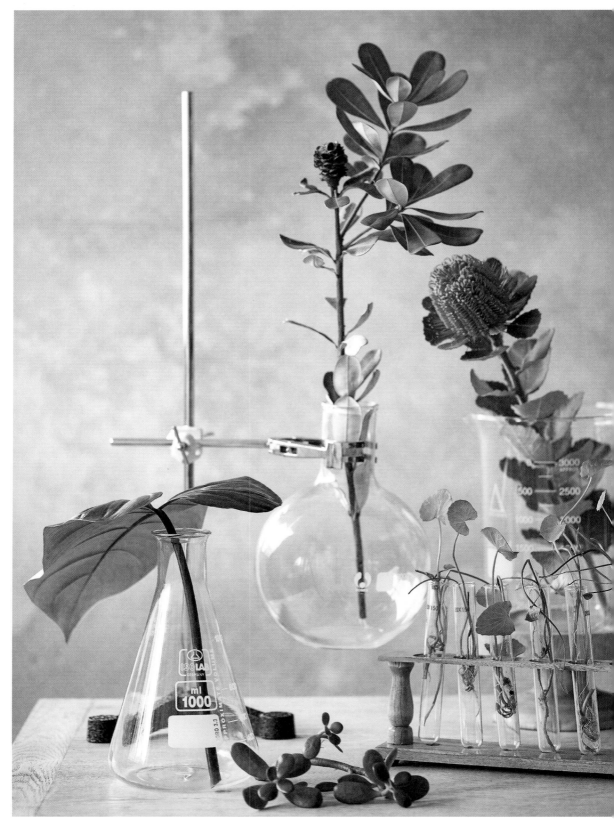

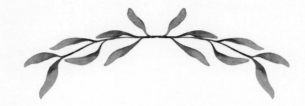

THE SUPPORTED GUT

Are you ready to romance and support your gut, learn its secret language and ways to care for it? Come with me to brush up on colon care, help decode well-used acronyms, and piece together where FODMAPS, SIBO and histamine intolerance fit in for you. Importantly, I'm going to show you how to use my GUTHEALS approach to deal with flare-ups and swiftly get your groove back.

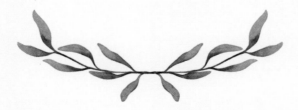

COLON CARE

Our current health climate is littered with detox diets, jumbled with juice cleanses and cluttered with colonics. Pull up a pew to discover how you can create a simple and natural toolkit for a clean and sparkling gut, and which cleansing foods can be used to boost colon health.

Three critical organs that help filter and clean up the body are the liver, which is your first line of defence; the kidneys, which continually filter your blood; and the colon, which is responsible for flushing out toxic waste.

It may not be the most glamorous part of the body, but we can't achieve thriving gut health without first acknowledging the colon. The mighty colon is your body's pipeline for waste removal, and to remain free from a build-up of pollutants and to experience real energy and vitality, we need to keep our colon in fighting shape to do its job as fuelling station and waste remover.

If your colon is burdened by digestive junk in your trunk, also known as toxic build-up and biofilm, you may experience symptoms of a sluggish colon, including:

- constipation
- bladder infections
- bad breath
- body odour
- digestive pain and cramping
- acne
- brain fog
- fatigue
- allergies
- poor sleep

In this case, eating a wholefoods diet high in lacto-fermenting bacteria will help to break through and release biofilm, clean out toxins, rebuild healthy gut flora and bring nourishment to the colon.

Keep the colon health boosters listed opposite in your gut health toolkit, and stay clean naturally without resorting to drastic measures.

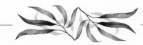

FOODS TO BOOST COLON HEALTH

- **CLOVES** and **FALSE BLACK PEPPER** (*Embelia ribes*) help break down biofilm.
- **APPLE CIDER VINEGAR** strips out the important minerals that help the biofilm matrix survive.
- High-therapeutic wholefood probiotics such as **COCONUT WATER KEFIR** and **COCONUT YOGHURT** can help rebuild healthy gut microbes quickly, which in turn will resynthesise nutrients from food, degrade toxins, and produce short-chain fatty acids to provide energy to the cells lining the colon.
- **FLAXSEEDS (LINSEEDS)**, **PSYLLIUM HUSKS** and **OATS** are high in plant-based fibre that help to sweep out the colon, increasing bowel movements and aiding detoxification.
- **CHLOROPHYLL-RICH FOODS** such as fresh green juices, wheatgrass, spinach, sprouts and dark leafy greens help soothe and heal damaged tissue in the colon, and draw out and carry toxins from the colon.
- Food-grade **DIATOMACEOUS EARTH** is a natural cleanser that helps lessen toxic build-up in the colon and remove heavy metals, also sweeping toxins, pathogenic bacteria and parasites from the body. A flavourless plant-based powder, it is made from the fossilised remains of diatoms, a type of hard-shelled algae, and can be added to smoothies, sprinkled on cereal or soups, or stirred into your morning porridge. I suggest starting with 1 teaspoon daily, building up slowly to 2 tablespoons a day. My Love Your Gut powder (see Appendix) is organic and the highest grade, best-quality product I've found.
- **WATER** is vital, so drink 2–3 litres (8–12 cups) of pure, filtered water per day to help keep your energy levels high, your cells happy and your gut hydrated and cleansed. A splash of lemon juice in warm water every morning is a great way to rehydrate and kick-start detoxification.

HOW TO IDENTIFY WHAT YOUR GUT IS TELLING YOU

The world of the digestive system is complex, and it's communicating with us all the time, but sometimes it's hard to know exactly what that 'gut feeling' is trying to tell us.

Cramps, bloating or other gut symptoms may be pointing to specific conditions or simple problems that have easy solutions. Always consult your GP or health practitioner if you're worried, otherwise the following signs may help decipher what your gut may be telling you.

SIGNS: Thrush, vaginal yeast infections, diarrhoea, flatulence, constipation, irritable bowel.
COULD BE: An overgrowth of the yeast *Candida albicans*.
TRY THIS: Seek diagnosis via a GP and do a stool test. Cut down on all sugar and processed food. Cut out all yeast from the diet, be kind to your gut and support it by eating probiotic-rich foods or taking a probiotic to restore healthy gut flora balance.

SIGNS: Bloating, cramps, loss of appetite, nausea, struggling to pass bowel movements.
COULD BE: Constipation.
TRY THIS: Increase intake of fibre-rich fruits and vegetables, take a few teaspoons of psyllium husks stirred into water twice a day, drink lots of filtered water and cut down on caffeine. Try gentle exercise such as walking or yoga to help digestion and increase bowel movements.

SIGNS: Pain in the tummy, side or mid- to lower back around the kidney area, and sometimes into the groin. Possible vomiting, loss of appetite, fever, shivering, diarrhoea, increased need to urinate, pain when urinating or blood in the urine.
COULD BE: Cystitis (urinary tract infection), kidney infection or kidney stones.
TRY THIS: See your GP immediately, drink lots of water and try a low-acid diet, which can help in the case of cystitis. Bicarbonate of soda (baking soda) also helps to temporarily alkalise the urine in your

bladder so it's less painful. Avoid scented soap, bubblebath and deodorant sprays as these will only make things worse. Natural bladder-soothing herbs taken as a tea can also help; try buchu, crataeva (*Craeteva nurvula*, also known as varuna) and uva ursi. Take garlic to help with the bacterial infection; echinacea, vitamin A, vitamin C and zinc also help your immune system.

SIGNS: Pain in the upper abdomen in a localised point. The pain is worse when the stomach is empty, which can wake you at night, and is eased by eating.
COULD BE: Gastritis (inflammation of the stomach lining), or a peptic ulcer (a sore within the lining of the stomach).
TRY THIS: If at any point the pain is accompanied by blood in the vomit or dark stools, call your local emergency services immediately, as this may be a bleeding ulcer. Otherwise consult a GP. Both conditions can be caused by overuse of anti-inflammatories, but can also be caused by an infection of *Helicobacter pylori*, which can be tested and treated by your doctor.

SIGNS: Urgently needing the loo, pain in the abdomen, abdominal distension (a look of being pregnant), changes in bowel movements including diarrhoea or constipation, bloating, excessive flatulence, fatigue, weakness and lethargy.
COULD BE: Irritable bowel syndrome, or possibly an inflammatory bowel disease or coeliac disease. Consult your GP.
TRY THIS: Immediately avoid rich fatty foods, high-fibre foods, caffeine and alcohol. Investigate with a health practitioner who can discover the cause and treatment; it might be that a FODMAP-friendly, SIBO or low-histamine diet could be one to try.

SIGNS: Frequent stomach cramps with nausea, vomiting and diarrhoea, combined with a high temperature and headaches.
COULD BE: Gastroenteritis (infectious diarrhoea).
TRY THIS: The most likely causes include food poisoning as a result of *Salmonella* or *Campylobacter* bacteria, or norovirus. If symptoms are severe, consult a GP immediately. In mild cases, hydrate by drinking lots of water with a pinch of Himalayan salt or Celtic sea salt, or coconut water.

Gut pain, as you can see, can be linked to a range of different conditions. However, if the cause of your symptoms is unclear, or sporadic, a great way to discover what could be happening within your gut is to keep a food diary. Writing down the foods you eat or drink over a two-week period, and noting any symptoms you feel after eating the meals, ranging from your energy levels through to specific symptoms or reactions, is a handy way to track how your gut is responding to foods.

It might take a couple of weeks for you to see a pattern of certain ingredients triggering particular responses. Once you've made any links to trigger foods you can take this information to a qualified health practitioner, and/or remove these foods for a period of time and see whether your symptoms disappear. My *Heal Your Gut* book and four-week Heal Your Gut online program can help you to understand and identify many of those trigger foods. You can find the information on my website, **superchargedfood.com**.

WHAT FLOATS YOUR BLOAT?

Ever felt, after eating a big dinner, like you're carrying a food baby that's due any minute? Has a muffin break at your desk had you fall straight into a food-induced coma? Do mysterious tummy aches and pains bother you after a particular meal? Read on ...

One of the common signs of poor gut health and digestion is bloating, noticeably after meals. If you experience bloating on a regular basis and feel like it has got out of hand, it could be a sign that something else is going on. Being bloated is not the same as carrying an extra tyre around your middle or being overweight.

There are many different reasons why your tummy is playing up — it could be related to a food allergy or intolerance, irregular bowel movements, overconsumption of inflammatory foods or artificial sweeteners, too much alcohol, certain medications, hormonal imbalances, indigestion, leaky gut, microbiome imbalances, or gastrointestinal disorders such as irritable bowel syndrome (IBS), coeliac disease, Crohn's disease or ulcerative colitis. IBS is common; research shows it affects around one-third of us, and despite almost 75 per cent of sufferers saying it severely impacts their work, relationships and sex lives, 60 per cent of those have never sought professional help due to embarrassment because of a poo taboo.[21]

Stress can also contribute to bloating, especially if you're someone who rushes out the door at breakfast, eats lunch while multi-tasking at a desk, then speeds through dinner between extracurricular activities.

Being bloated is most often a result of gas and wind trapped in your digestive system, which makes your stomach protrude, your waistband become tighter and your digestion sluggish. This can arise due to inadequate protein digestion, where some foods remain in the gut and start to ferment, or an inability to fully break down sugars and other carbohydrates if you're lacking in digestive enzymes, or imbalances in gut bacteria.

For many, bloating comes and goes and is temporary, but if your bloating is associated with other signs — such as a fever, skin rashes or hives, watery eyes, itchy throat and other signs of allergic reaction, constipation or diarrhoea, vomiting or nausea, blood in your urine or stool, brain fog and difficulty concentrating, irregular periods, unintentional weight loss, trouble going to the bathroom, pain around your lymph nodes (including in your groin, throat or armpits), or heavy fatigue — then it's best to consult your GP to find out if there's an underlying health issue causing your bloating.

Let's look at a few of the lifestyle and dietary issues that may also be floating your bloat.

LOOK OUT FOR STRESS AND NEGATIVE EMOTION

Your gut is very sensitive to what's going on in your life mentally and emotionally. Negative emotions and stress are two of the biggest triggers for an upset tummy. Generally, when we find ourselves in a specific stressful situation (a work deadline, an argument with a partner) we're aware of the tension, both physically and mentally.

But sometimes, the stress or negativity goes unnoticed or is unconsciously buried deep in our subconscious to protect us from the pain and discomfort. When this happens, your bloating becomes a way for your body to communicate with you.

Are you feeling overwhelmed? Are you holding on to emotions, such as fear and anger, and accumulating them instead of 'digesting' them? Take some time to look honestly at what's going on in your life on a deeper level, rather than just the sort of foods you're eating.

There might be a very powerful message behind your bloating that you're currently unaware of.

BE PRESENT WHILE YOU EAT

When you're feeling stressed, upset or rushed, your nervous system goes into fight-or-flight mode. Stress hormones are high and blood flow to your gut is reduced, which makes your digestion slower.

When you're stressed, as food is not properly digested, fermentation and bloating can occur. To avoid this, always eat in a quiet environment and try to eat 'mindfully'.

Sit down and take a few deep belly breaths. Never eat standing, at your desk, or while checking your phone. To give your digestive system all the support it needs to optimally digest your food, be mindful of the food you're eating and the amazing process happening inside your body.

Start by thoroughly chewing your food. We've all heard that digestion starts in the mouth, yet very few of us chew our food properly. This advice alone could greatly reduce your bloating. Slow down when you're chewing your food and enjoy the taste and flavours on your palate.

Eat slowly and put your fork down after each bite. Eating quickly causes more air to be sucked into your stomach, resulting in gas and bloating.

After implementing these strategies you'll begin to notice positive changes in your digestion. But if you still have uncomfortable symptoms, try avoiding these other common causes.

AVOID CHEWING GUM

Chewing gum leads to swallowing air, which can cause bloating. Plus, sugar-free gums are usually packed with sugar alcohol, such as mannitol, sorbitol and xylitol, which are notorious for causing gas.

DON'T GUZZLE OR DRINK THROUGH A STRAW

I'm a fierce advocate of listening to your body cues, so I'll never encourage you to not drink if you're thirsty. However, try to avoid gulping down large amounts of water while eating, as it will dilute your digestive enzymes, making your digestion weaker and bloating more likely to occur. Drink at least 30 minutes before eating.

The pre-digestive recipes on pages 146–149 of this book will help to strengthen your digestion.

There's an old Chinese proverb that says, 'It's better to eat a rock sitting down than a meal standing up.' I like to remember this when I'm feeling rushed or on the go, as it makes me smile and reminds me to take the time to sit and eat properly and be more thoughtful around meal times.

DON'T EAT FRUIT AT THE END OF A MEAL

Fruit is digested very quickly — much faster than anything else, especially animal protein, dairy and grains. If you like to eat fruit, try enjoying it on an empty stomach instead: first thing in the morning, or as a mid-morning or mid-afternoon snack.

AVOID PROCESSED FOODS

Processed and packaged foods — 'frankenfoods' — are full of chemicals, preservatives, dyes and other ingredients that our digestive systems don't know how to process.

Gums and thickeners (carrageenan, xanthan gum and guar gum, in particular), are hidden everywhere, especially in protein bars, and can cause gastrointestinal distress because they alter the balance of gut flora and are highly fermentable.

There are many other potential causes for your bloating, such as food intolerances, candida, SIBO (small intestine bacterial overgrowth) and parasites. But before you spend your time and money on blood, stool, breath and urine tests, I invite you to try the simple tips above and look at your bloating from a different perspective. They might just help you say bye bye to that food baby forever — and let's face it, we all want to fit comfortably into our favourite pants and do the top button up!

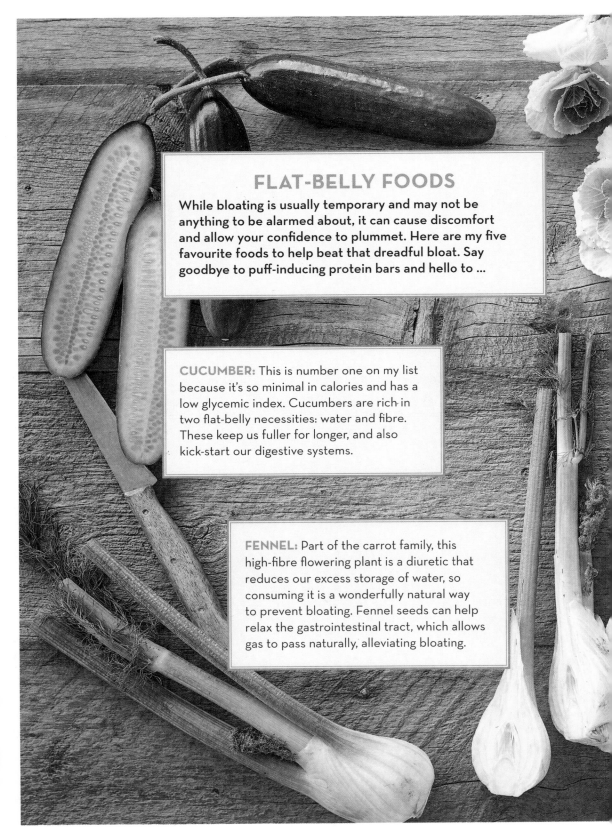

FLAT-BELLY FOODS

While bloating is usually temporary and may not be anything to be alarmed about, it can cause discomfort and allow your confidence to plummet. Here are my five favourite foods to help beat that dreadful bloat. Say goodbye to puff-inducing protein bars and hello to ...

CUCUMBER: This is number one on my list because it's so minimal in calories and has a low glycemic index. Cucumbers are rich in two flat-belly necessities: water and fibre. These keep us fuller for longer, and also kick-start our digestive systems.

FENNEL: Part of the carrot family, this high-fibre flowering plant is a diuretic that reduces our excess storage of water, so consuming it is a wonderfully natural way to prevent bloating. Fennel seeds can help relax the gastrointestinal tract, which allows gas to pass naturally, alleviating bloating.

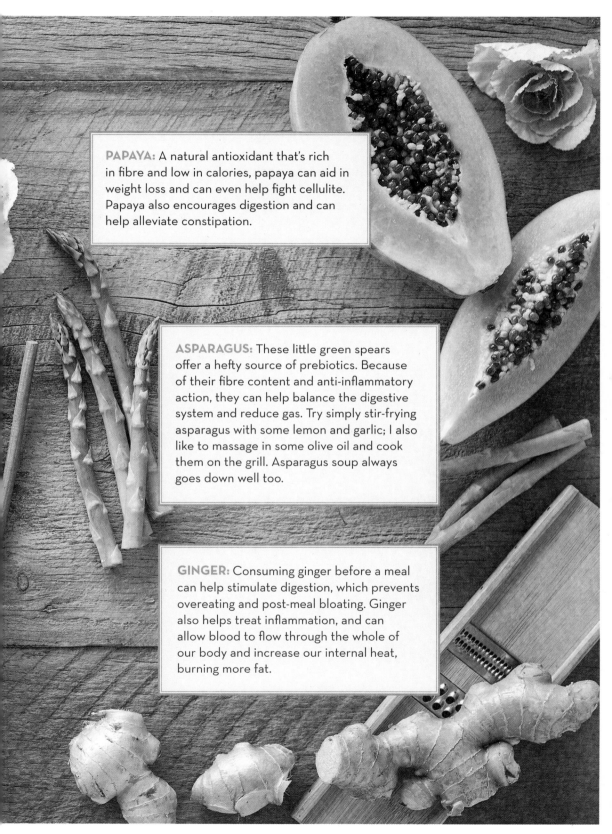

PAPAYA: A natural antioxidant that's rich in fibre and low in calories, papaya can aid in weight loss and can even help fight cellulite. Papaya also encourages digestion and can help alleviate constipation.

ASPARAGUS: These little green spears offer a hefty source of prebiotics. Because of their fibre content and anti-inflammatory action, they can help balance the digestive system and reduce gas. Try simply stir-frying asparagus with some lemon and garlic; I also like to massage in some olive oil and cook them on the grill. Asparagus soup always goes down well too.

GINGER: Consuming ginger before a meal can help stimulate digestion, which prevents overeating and post-meal bloating. Ginger also helps treat inflammation, and can allow blood to flow through the whole of our body and increase our internal heat, burning more fat.

WHERE DO FODMAPS FIT IN?

For people with irritable bowel syndrome (IBS), a low-FODMAP diet can be especially helpful. Many people with IBS are unable to absorb certain molecules in food, which can lead to gut issues such as gas, bloating, diarrhoea and constipation. The FODMAP diet was pioneered by a team at Monash University, led by Professor Peter Gibson and including Dr Sue Shepherd and others.

FODMAP STANDS FOR ...

Fermentable: meaning they are broken down (fermented) by bacteria in the large bowel, and not absorbed in the small intestine

Oligosaccharides: more complex sugars, such as fructans and galacto-oligosaccharides

Disaccharides: 'double' sugar molecules, such as lactose

Monosaccharides: single sugars, such as fructose

And Polyols: sugar alcohols, such as sorbitol, mannitol, maltitol and xylitol; isomalt and polydextrose act in a similar way.

Essentially, these molecules, when poorly absorbed by our small intestine, move into our large intestine, where our good bacteria ferment them. This process of fermentation leads to IBS symptoms — enter gas and bloating.

The FODMAP diet isn't a 'one size fits all' approach — so while there are plenty of resources online, simply visiting Dr Google for a list of FODMAP-friendly foods often leads to more confusion as to what you actually can or cannot eat. Some people can happily eat polyol molecules but categorically no disaccharides; others cannot eat either of these.

To ensure the Supercharge Your Gut maintenance program is FODMAP- friendly you'll want to step away from foods containing the ingredients that irritate you. Fruits and vegetables will be the main areas that need switching. IBS sufferers may find eating large amounts of fruit and vegetables and fibre upsets their gut, either because they have a laxative effect, or because the fibre in the skin is too harsh.

As a rule of thumb, garlic and onion are the main culprits, which can be replaced with the green tops of the spring onion (scallion) to add the allium flavour to your meals, or the Indian herb asafoetida, or you can use an infused olive oil.

If the FODMAP diet seems too daunting, just remember, FODMAPs are forms of carbohydrates, so if all else fails, just make a few tweaks and remember that good fats are your friend.

And if your neighbour with the gorgeous glowing skin swears by chia seeds in her smoothies, yet when you add them you feel bloated, take heed — your body is trying to tell you something. Open a direct phone line to your body and it will give you the answers.

WHAT IF I'M VEGETARIAN?

No problem! You just need to think about eating adequate foods full of nutrients from non-meat sources to ensure you're supporting your body fully. The Supercharge Your Gut program is filled with plenty of nutrient-dense meal options that are fantastic for vegetarians, but it's crucial to incorporate foods high in protein, iron and vitamin B12 each week.

POWER UP ON PROTEIN

Dietary proteins are an important part of a balanced diet, and not just for buff body builders. They have a significant impact on gut health, as they serve as the major source of nitrogen for colonic microbial growth, and are essential for the absorption of carbohydrates and production of beneficial products within the gut.[22]

It's vital to consume a wide range of good-quality protein sources, to ensure your diet contains all nine essential amino acids — the ones the body cannot manufacture.

There are lots of simple ways to ramp up your protein intake.

- Add ½ cup of quinoa to soups.
- Choose protein-rich vegetables such as green peas, broccoli, artichokes and leafy greens.
- Add spirulina to smoothies.
- Use nut milk for smoothies — almond, cashew and pistachio milks are highest in protein.
- Add a sprinkle of chia seeds to desserts and smoothies.
- Add hemp powder or seeds to smoothies (if legally available).
- If you can tolerate them after the first few weeks, start to add high-protein lentils, chickpeas, white beans or pinto beans to soups. First soak the legumes overnight and rinse them, so they're easier

to digest; adding kombu (dried seaweed) to the cooking water also makes them easier on the tummy, and their nutrients more bioavailable.

THE IMPORTANCE OF VITAMIN B12

Vitamin B12 has a wide range of health benefits including supporting the heart, brain and nervous system, producing energy and improving mood. It plays a major role in the production of digestive enzymes and is needed to break down foods in the stomach. It also helps foster healthy bacteria within the gut environment, and eliminate the harmful bacteria within the digestive tract. A B12 deficiency can affect the nervous system, which includes reducing the nerve transmissions to the gastrointestinal tract, resulting in digestive issues such as constipation.[23]

Vitamin B12 is almost exclusively found in animal products such as red meats, poultry and seafood, so it's important for vegetarians to include foods such as organic free-range eggs, nutritional yeast, and nut milks or coconut milk that are fortified with B12.

IRON — AND HOW TO GET IT

Another essential dietary mineral is iron, which is involved in various bodily functions including energy production and immune support. Vegetarian diets are generally high enough in iron from plant-based foods; the issue lies in the absorption of the iron.

There are two types of iron — haem iron, which is found in animal foods; and non-haem iron, found in plants. Vegetarian food sources high in iron include quinoa, green leafy vegetables, nuts, seeds and eggs. If nuts are hard for you to digest, try drinking nut milks or adding nut butter to smoothies. Non-haem iron is not absorbed as easily as haem iron, but there are genius ways you can increase your iron absorption.

- Eating smaller amounts of iron-rich food more frequently will increase the absorption.
- Absorption increases by five times when non-haem iron is consumed with foods rich in vitamin C, so simply adding a squeeze of lemon to your foods can increase iron absorption.
- Tea and coffee addicts, listen up. These drinks (even decaf!) contain tannins that inhibit iron absorption — so avoid consuming them around the same time as iron-rich foods.
- Diatomaceous earth powder (see page 43) is rich in absorbable iron.

THE CLEANSING GREEN MINESTRONE on (page 223) is a glorious addition to a vegetarian diet — containing iron-rich dark leafy greens, served with nutritional yeast for vitamin B12, and a squeeze of lemon for extra iron absorption, thanks to its vitamin C. You can also add ½ cup of quinoa for extra protein, ensuring you have covered four essential nutrients in four easy steps.

UNDERSTANDING SIBO

To get down to specifics, your gut microbiome lives throughout your entire digestive tract, but in varied amounts depending on the location. Only a small number of bacteria live within the small instestine compared to other regions — with only around 10,000 bacteria per millilitre of fluid, as opposed to 1,000,000,000 per millilitre in the large intestine or colon.

Depending on the area of the gut, the strains of bacteria present are also different. The small intestine is dependent on specific numbers and specific types of bacteria, and for good reason: it's an important area for absorption of nutrients, fighting off infections and regulating the immune system, thanks to its impressive army of lymphoid cells.

Within a normal, healthy small intestine, a balance of beneficial organisms works as a team to protect against yeasts and pathogenic bacteria, and produce important nutrients such as vitamin K, folate and short-chain fatty acids. They also help you to maintain normal muscular activity within the colon, which keeps you regular.

SIBO (small intestinal bacterial overgrowth) occurs when there's an increase in the number of bacteria present in the small intestine, and an overgrowth within the small intestine of certain strains of bacteria that should normally live within the colon.

Why is this a bad thing? For starters, SIBO negatively affects the structure of the small intestine, which can affect the way your nutrients are absorbed by damaging the cells of your gut. This damage can also lead to leaky gut — where the intestinal wall becomes permeable to proteins, which then make their way into the bloodstream. This can cause abnormal immune responses, allergies, intolerances and autoimmune diseases.

The unwanted bacteria present in the case of SIBO will also take up important vitamins, such as B12, before your body can absorb them. They can also steal protein and amino acids, and affect the absorption of important fats and fat-soluble vitamins such as A and D.

SYMPTOMS OF SIBO INCLUDE:

- weight loss and nutrient deficiencies
- abdominal pain and discomfort
- bloating after meals
- gas
- diarrhoea
- abdominal distension
- food intolerances or allergies

If you suffer from any of these common associated conditions, you can check if you have SIBO with a simple breath test, which you can order online, or do through your GP or health practitioner.

Diet plays a major role in helping to eradicate SIBO and prevent relapse. A combination of low-FODMAP, low-sugar and Supercharge Your Gut principles are effective in rebalancing the gut to a healthy state.

COULD I HAVE HISTAMINE INTOLERANCE?

When you're trying to heal your gut from a lifetime's worth of mistreatment — whether from use of antibiotics, incorrect diet, disease, stress or a combination of these — it can be really frustrating when all your dietary changes fail to improve your varied, unpleasant symptoms.

Headaches, bowel irregularities, fatigue, energy depletion, skin eruptions such as hives and rashes, acne, food intolerances — all these symptoms could be the result of many underlying conditions, and it can be hard to know where to even start when pinning down the true culprit.

If you're one of those people who has explored every other protocol under the sun, but you're still experiencing the same symptoms, a histamine intolerance may possibly be the missing link. In this case, giving a low-histamine diet a try might offer the answers you've been searching for.

Histamines are neurotransmitters that are triggered during an allergic reaction. These act as an alert to the immune system, causing an instant inflammatory response to protect the body from foreign invaders. Histamines are a clever way of your body communicating to your brain when something enters your body that shouldn't be there, and results in the puffy eyes or swollen lips or hives that may require you to obtain antihistamine drugs from a doctor or pharmacist.

Importantly from a gut health perspective, histamines can also be absorbed from histamine-containing foods.

In normal circumstances, the body will balance out histamine production with an enzyme called diamine oxidase (DAO), which prevents the over-accumulation of histamines within the body.

The biggest non-food source of histamines in most of us is our gut flora. While certain types of bacteria produce histamines, others degrade them. Too many histamine-producing bacteria can cause our system to build up histamine levels faster than our DAO enzyme can remove them.

The mucosal lining of our digestive tract also produces DAO, and if the lining is irritated, DAO production also decreases.

Nutritionally, magnesium-rich foods can help; low-histamine options include green leafy vegetables, oatmeal, beans, flaxseeds (linseeds), almonds, fresh salmon (not tinned), coriander (cilantro), basil and cumin, or you could even try a magnesium supplement. As magnesium can be hard to absorb via the gut, and gut issues make absorption even harder, a topical magnesium spray is a good option.

As with most dietary issues, individual sensitivities vary significantly, and most people only have trouble with the very high-histamine foods. In addition, histamine reactions occur when histamines slowly build up in the body, so having the trigger foods now and then is fine for many people. It's only when histamine levels have risen to a certain point that symptoms suddenly erupt, which is when dietary changes can bring it all back into balance.

During the Supercharge Your Gut protocol, you can ditch certain foods that are high in histamines. When making the recipes, apply the low-histamine options shown on the next page, and consume probiotic and prebiotic foods such as chicory root, leek, asparagus and artichoke.

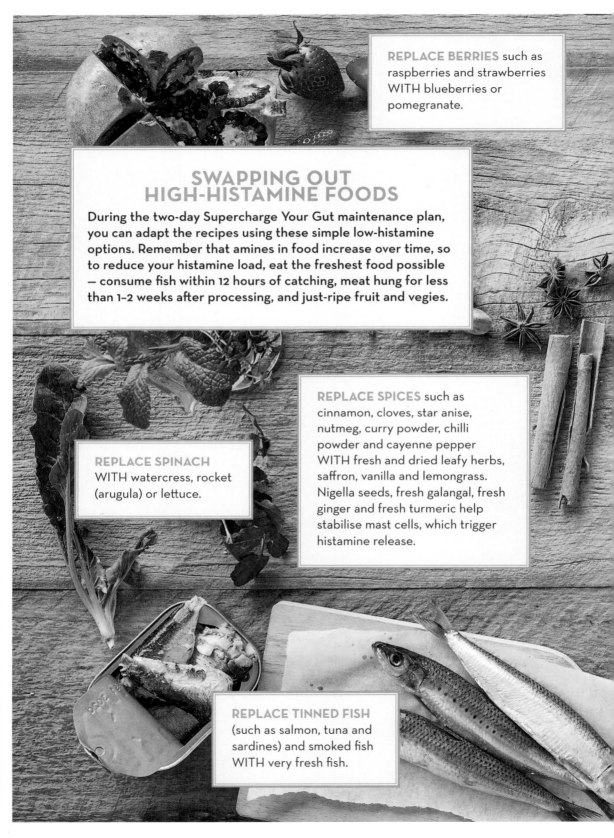

REPLACE BERRIES such as raspberries and strawberries WITH blueberries or pomegranate.

SWAPPING OUT HIGH-HISTAMINE FOODS

During the two-day Supercharge Your Gut maintenance plan, you can adapt the recipes using these simple low-histamine options. Remember that amines in food increase over time, so to reduce your histamine load, eat the freshest food possible — consume fish within 12 hours of catching, meat hung for less than 1–2 weeks after processing, and just-ripe fruit and vegies.

REPLACE SPICES such as cinnamon, cloves, star anise, nutmeg, curry powder, chilli powder and cayenne pepper WITH fresh and dried leafy herbs, saffron, vanilla and lemongrass. Nigella seeds, fresh galangal, fresh ginger and fresh turmeric help stabilise mast cells, which trigger histamine release.

REPLACE SPINACH WITH watercress, rocket (arugula) or lettuce.

REPLACE TINNED FISH (such as salmon, tuna and sardines) and smoked fish WITH very fresh fish.

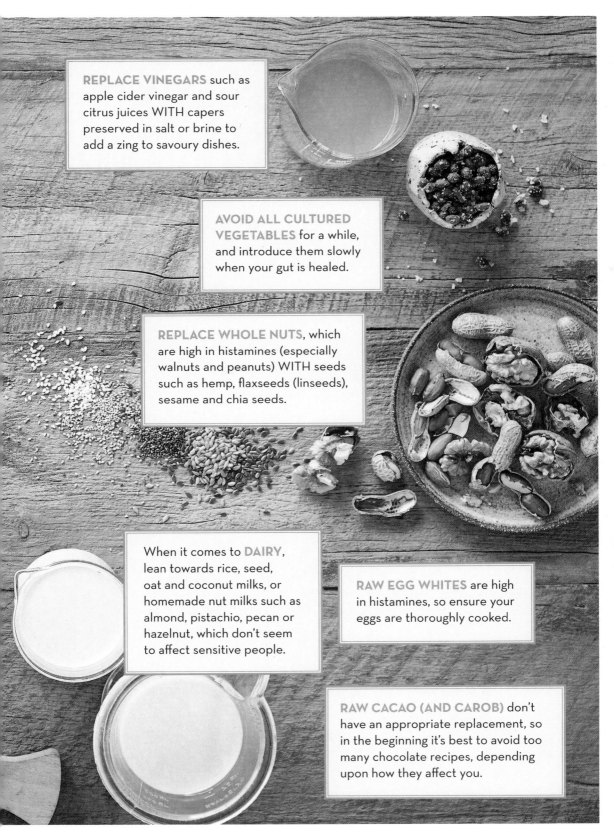

REPLACE VINEGARS such as apple cider vinegar and sour citrus juices **WITH** capers preserved in salt or brine to add a zing to savoury dishes.

AVOID ALL CULTURED VEGETABLES for a while, and introduce them slowly when your gut is healed.

REPLACE WHOLE NUTS, which are high in histamines (especially walnuts and peanuts) **WITH** seeds such as hemp, flaxseeds (linseeds), sesame and chia seeds.

When it comes to **DAIRY**, lean towards rice, seed, oat and coconut milks, or homemade nut milks such as almond, pistachio, pecan or hazelnut, which don't seem to affect sensitive people.

RAW EGG WHITES are high in histamines, so ensure your eggs are thoroughly cooked.

RAW CACAO (AND CAROB) don't have an appropriate replacement, so in the beginning it's best to avoid too many chocolate recipes, depending upon how they affect you.

DEALING WITH FLARE-UPS

A gut flare-up can stop you in your tracks. If you experience one, this is your body screaming out to you to take it easy, slow down and to move into 'rest and digest' mode.

If you've ever had an upset stomach, you may have been referred to the BRAT (bananas, rice, applesauce, toast) diet, which is touted as a gentle, easy-to-digest style of eating. However, I'm not convinced that these four ingredients are necessarily easy to digest for everybody — particularly in instances of autoimmunity, leaky gut or candida, where bad bacteria will have a field day when that feast of carbohydrates enters their territory.

If we're really going to truly rest and digest, then we need nourish the gut through wholefoods that soothe the gut wall, and are low in sugars and high in anti-inflammatory ingredients.

The BRAT approach is aimed at firming up stools, using bland, low-fibre and starchy 'binding' foods that will help in the case of diarrhoea. But the BRAT diet won't be so helpful if your flare-up is connected to symptoms of constipation.

While bananas are great for replacing nutrients lost during diarrhoea, there are other supercharged ingredients that are also wonderful for nourishing your gut during a flare-up, and denser in nutrients and healing qualities than starchy toast and rice.

- Plantain is like a less sugary banana that requires cooking. It's a great addition or replacement for bananas in the BRAT diet, offering more vitamins A and C, zinc, magnesium and potassium. (Check out my delicious plantain chips, opposite.)
- Butternut squash is a great starch substitute for rice and toast, offering 350–435 per cent of the daily requirement for vitamin A, which is lost in cases of diarrhoea and vomiting. Squash has more potassium than bananas, and also provides vitamin C, manganese, magnesium, and the B vitamins folate, thiamine, niacin and pantothenic acid.

For condition-specific flare-ups, you can try the approach outlined on pages 62–63 — but always consult your medical practitioner if you're worried or if symptoms persist. The GUTHEALS approach (see pages 64–65) will also help to boost the immune system during a flare-up.

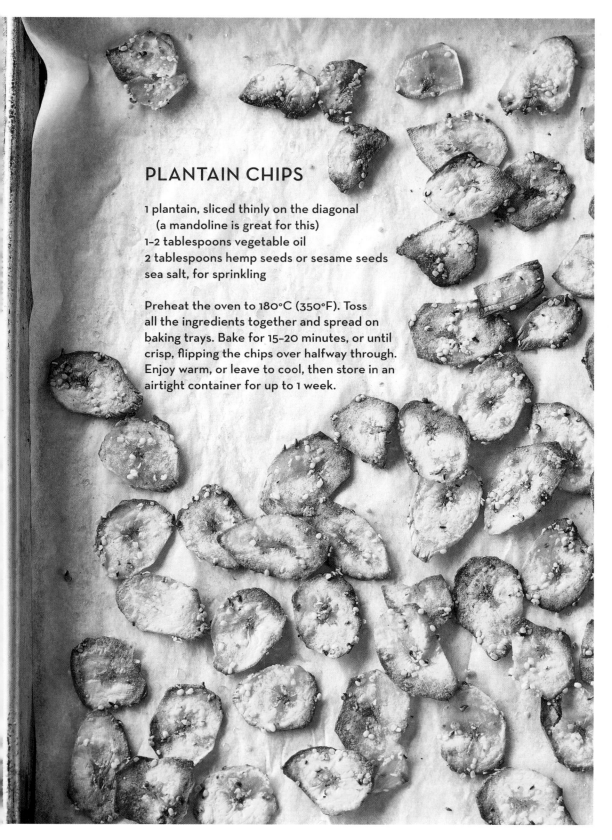

PLANTAIN CHIPS

1 plantain, sliced thinly on the diagonal
  (a mandoline is great for this)
1–2 tablespoons vegetable oil
2 tablespoons hemp seeds or sesame seeds
sea salt, for sprinkling

Preheat the oven to 180°C (350°F). Toss
all the ingredients together and spread on
baking trays. Bake for 15–20 minutes, or until
crisp, flipping the chips over halfway through.
Enjoy warm, or leave to cool, then store in an
airtight container for up to 1 week.

- **DIARRHOEA:** Consume plenty of fluids, including filtered water, and herbal teas such as chamomile or peppermint to soothe the digestive tract. Add a pinch of Himalayan salt to water, or drink 100 per cent coconut water to help replace electrolytes that may have been lost. Bone broths hydrate and supply soothing gelatine to the gut.

- **CONSTIPATION:** Avoid gluten-containing grains, as these contain sticky proteins known as prolamins, which will back you up even more. Make smoothies with chia seeds, berries and avocados, which are all high in fibre. Vegetables such as broccoli and brussels sprouts, onions, sweet potatoes, cauliflower and green beans are excellent foods high in soluble and insoluble fibre to help move things along, if you can tolerate them without becoming bloated. Drink more water, reduce your sugar load, and increase your intake of probiotic-rich foods. Organic black coffee can also help to soften your stools.

- **CROHN'S DISEASE AND ULCERATIVE COLITIS:** These are inflammatory conditions, and for flare-ups involving diarrhoea you should try the diarrhoea recommendations above. Drink loads of fluids including broths and chamomile tea, which is soothing. Turmeric tea is highly anti-inflammatory, and consuming oily fish such as sardines, salmon and tuna will supply anti-inflammatory oils. During a flare-up, avoid grains and artificial sweeteners, and say hello to pure aloe vera juice. Avoid seeds, nuts, vegetable and fruit skins, excessive fibre, artificial ingredients and additives, coffee and alcohol.

- **COELIAC DISEASE:** Avoid all gluten. Eat plain foods: meats and vegetables are a safe bet. Oily fish will be anti-inflammatory and calming to the gut. Sleep and rest as much as possible. Consume bone broth regularly and employ stress-lowering practices such as deep breathing and relaxation techniques.

- **IRRITABLE BOWEL SYNDROME (IBS):** Consume psyllium, which is an adaptogenic fibre — it will increase bowel movement or decrease it, depending on what your body needs. Eat more fermented foods to increase good bacteria; avoid sugar to control the bad microbial communities. Take a few tablespoons of organic flaxseed (linseed) meal a day. Address emotional issues by writing in a journal, or practise positive affirmations and meditation.

- **LEAKY GUT:** Bone broth, bone broth, bone broth! This is so important to calm and soothe the gut wall. Avoid gluten and grains. Focus on soups and stews, or slowly cooked meats and vegetables, which are easy to digest. If you're ready for it and it doesn't give you bloating or pain, consume fermented vegetables and coconut yoghurt or coconut water kefir, which will help to recolonise the gut and increase immunity.

- **HEARTBURN AND ACID REFLUX:** Avoid stimulating foods such as caffeine, chilli and chocolate, which can exacerbate symptoms. Consume fermented vegetables and increase stomach acid through ingredients such as Himalayan salt and apple cider vinegar. Consume ginger tea and chamomile tea, which have a gastro-protective effect. Pour 500 ml (17 fl oz/2 cups) boiling water over 4 g (about 2 tablespoons) of powdered slippery elm bark, then steep for 3–5 minutes; drink three times per day.

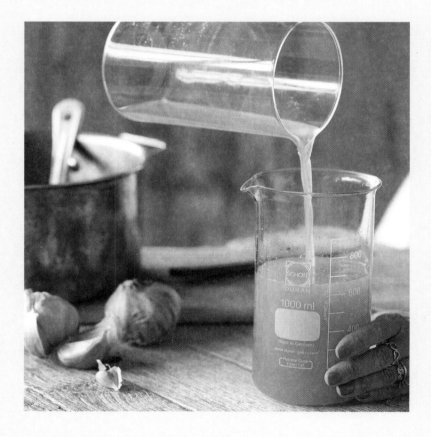

THE GUTHEALS APPROACH

For non-specific conditions, or for an all-round gut flare-up protocol, try my GUTHEALS approach, which is an alternative to the BRAT diet and will help across a range of flare-ups. When nothing else will really work, this will cover all the bases until you've spoken to your health professional. Begin with the following ...

- Ginger and garlic in teas or drinks.
- Unsweetened coconut yoghurt for probiotics.
- Turmeric for its potent anti-inflammatory effects.
- Herbal remedies such as slippery elm, marshmallow root and deglycyrrhizinated liquorice to repair the lining of the gut.
- Eggs, scrambled or poached.
- Aloe vera, juice or gummies (see page 276).
- Liquid meals such as bone broths, smoothies and puréed soups, which are much easier on the gastrointestinal tract and can help to reduce the pain of a flare, bloating and indigestion.
- Salmon and oily fish — or if vegetarian, flaxseeds (linseeds) — for omega-3s, once symptoms settle down.

The GUTHEALS protocol should be employed immediately at the first sign of a flare-up, and followed for three to five days.

Here are some important and helpful things to note when applying the GUTHEALS approach.

- STAY HYDRATED: Replace lost body fluids during a flare-up of vomiting or diarrhoea by prioritising hydration before all else. Start by sipping small amounts of water every five minutes. Consider drinking water from a fresh young coconut, which is high in electrolytes. You can also try medicinal teas such as peppermint, chamomile, peppermint or fennel, which are ultra-soothing for the gut. And your number-one best friend during GUTHEALS is broth! Drink a couple of mugs a day.
- FOCUS COMPLETELY on cooked, warm foods, and hold the ice in those smoothies. Cooking will provide the heat needed to help break down the tough cell walls of raw foods, making them much easier to digest.

- **REST AND DIGEST!** Take the time to really rest and have the convalescence you need to recover. Put your feet up, take some time off, say no to unnecessary commitments. This is a time when you need to heal and put your gut-healthy principles into practice.
- **AFTER TWO TO THREE DAYS**, if all symptoms have subsided, you can do a test at slowly reintroducing your regular diet. If this provokes any reactions or flare-ups again, this might be a good sign to consult a qualified naturopath or integrative GP to see how to best move forward with your unique situation.

After the first couple of days, to ease back into normal eating, a typical day might include the following ideas.

- **EARLY MORNING:** A raw chopped garlic clove taken with 1 litre (35 fl oz/4 cups) filtered water.
- **BREAKFAST:** Smoothie based on coconut milk and coconut yoghurt with berries, flaxseeds (linseeds) and slippery elm (or other gut-healing herbs).
- **MORNING TEA:** Fresh turmeric and ginger tea followed by a shot of aloe vera juice (or a homemade Aloe Vera Gummy, page 276).
- **LUNCH:** Scrambled eggs with wilted spinach, followed by a cup of bone broth.
- **AFTERNOON TEA:** A cup of homemade puréed vegetable soup.
- **DINNER:** Salmon with roasted pumpkin (squash), and plantains fried in coconut oil.

Look up at the sky and imagine that there are a thousand times as many bacteria in your gut as there are stars in the Milky Way — 100 trillion vs 100 billion.

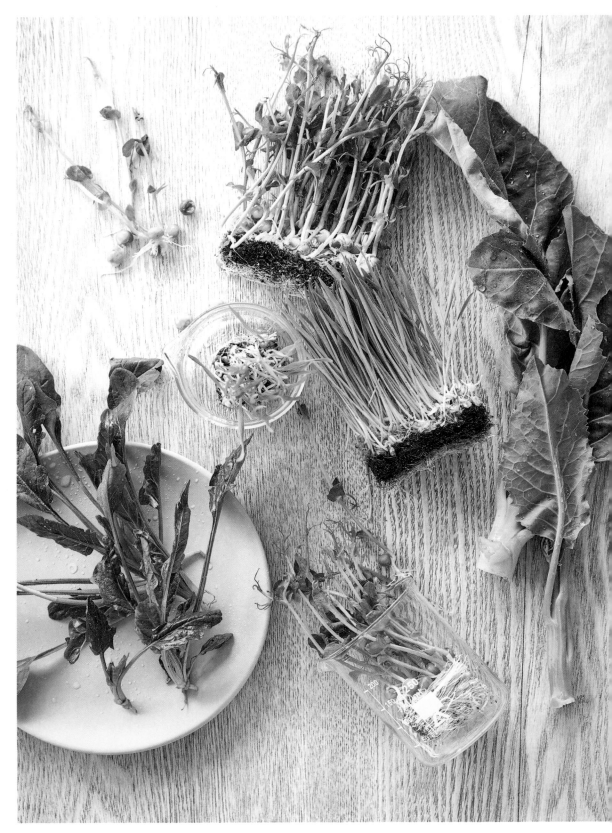

THE WELL-FED GUT

*You know that your digestive system can 'talk',
so what is it saying to you right now?
Is there a disturbance in the force? Perhaps
it's fed up with working overtime in a messed-up
system, or in a stitch about unusual trigger foods
that have sent it into a tailspin?*

*A well-fed gut means eating for digestibility,
repairing the gut lining, and feeding and
replenishing your microbiome with
gut-friendly foods.*

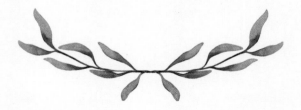

EATING FOR DIGESTIBILITY

When seeking to attain a desired level of health, it's common to focus on the nutritional properties of foods — but what about the digestibility of our food, particularly if our gut has been compromised in any way?

We are showered with conflicting information about what to eat. Many 'raw food' advocates believe food is best eaten in its natural unprepared state, with all the enzymes intact, and that this is better for us nutritionally, which can often be the case — but for a person with compromised gut health, raw foods can be very hard to digest. In traditional Chinese medicine, raw foods are considered too *yin* or 'cold' in nature, placing a damper on our digestive fire.

Consuming hard-to-digest foods over long periods can add a real burden to the gut lining, by wearing down our epithelial cells and microvilli, and the enzymes they produce; these enzymes digest carbohydrates, fats and proteins effectively, without damaging or irritating the lining of the gut.

Eating foods that are easy to digest is a crucial step in creating an environment in which our epithelial cells are free to do the complex job of digestion so our body can uptake nutrients and function at its peak.

It was only once I let go of salads that my gut healing truly began; for me, it was a 'light bulb' moment, and really showed the difference that cooked and pre-digestible foods could make to my health, and particularly my energy levels.

If you're not sure which foods to embrace and avoid on your Supercharged Gut days, follow this simple guide.

FOODS TO AVOID

- Say 'pasta la vista baby' to white starchy carbohydrates (white rice, pasta, crackers, commercial breads, cakes), confectionery and sweets, and foods with artificial ingredients and additives.
- Give deep-fried or fatty foods the flick.
- Say no to genetically modified foods.
- Leave high-gluten foods such as wheat, barley and triticale on the shelf.
- Say so long to unsoaked or unsprouted grains.

- Leave large amounts of unactivated nuts, and nut meal flours that haven't been pre-soaked and dehydrated, to the squirrels.
- Watch out for excessive meat consumption.
- Untangle yourself from unfermented pasteurised dairy, such as low-fat milk.
- Avoid an excess of raw foods, especially crucifers such as kale and cabbage, and vegetables such as chard.

FOODS TO EMBRACE

For digestibility, enjoy foods that are gentle on the gut and have a healing, anti-inflammatory effect.

- COOKED FOODS: Lightly steaming, sautéing, stewing or roasting vegetables and slow-cooking meats enables the cell walls and/or membranes of these foods to be gently broken down, releasing maximum nutrition in an easy-to-digest form.
- BONE BROTHS: These are high in minerals and gelatine, which is supportive of the gut and improves protein digestibility.
- SPROUTED, SOAKED OR FERMENTED GLUTEN-FREE GRAINS, NUTS AND SEEDS: Proper preparation breaks down the enzyme and mineral inhibitors that irritate the gut and prevent nutrient uptake. Although raw nuts can be taxing on the gut, some people can tolerate nut butters well, and I've included these in the recipes.
- FERMENTED FOODS: In small amounts, with meals, cultured foods including full-fat organic yoghurt and kefir, and cultured vegetables such as sauerkraut and kimchi, are easy to digest and create a healthy inner ecology, as well as providing enzymes to help break down other foods.
- EXTRA VIRGIN COCONUT OIL: Contains medium-chain fatty acids that are easier to digest than other fats, and that promote healthy species of gut bacteria and ward off harmful microbes.
- EXTRA VIRGIN OLIVE OIL: Highly anti-inflammatory and helps keep things moving in the bowel.
- FIBRE-RICH FOODS: Sprouted seeds and lightly cooked vegetables are your best sources.
- OMEGA-3 FATTY ACIDS: Small amounts from flaxseed oil, sustainable fish oils and activated walnuts or walnut oil will provide anti-inflammatory benefits to keep the gut healthy.

- **FRUITS:** Berries, prunes, figs, ripe bananas and avocados are easy to digest and gentle on the gut.
- **VEGETABLES:** Your most easily digestible garden dwellers are zucchini (courgette), sweet potato, cucumber, carrot, lettuce, pumpkin (squash), parsnip, beetroot (beet) and turnip, as they are lower in insoluble fibre than other vegetables.
- **SOUPS, SMOOTHIES AND SLURPIES:** Blending wholesome, gut-friendly foods increases their gentleness on the digestive system. Because the fibres are so finely broken down, they take a huge burden off the gut, and their nutrients are absorbed more efficiently. Consider the blending process an external form of digestion. But don't forget to 'chew' your smoothie. Liquids should still be allowed the time to combine with saliva in the mouth, as this is the first vital step in the digestion process.

IDENTIFYING TRIGGER FOODS

If you're having gut issues, I'd like to suggest that you consider the idea of a food-elimination trial, not as a torturous ordeal depriving you of all your favourite foods, but as a sensible and sustainable approach that reframes your food choices by 'checking in' with your body and how it responds to different foods in different seasons and stages.

The aim is to reduce inflammation, and to be aware of and record inflammatory responses in a food diary, especially in the initial few weeks. Inflammatory responses to a food may include sore back, aching joints, bloating, tiredness, abdominal pain, throat irritation, coughing or sneezing after eating, mood problems, headaches or migraines, itchiness, mucus, a foggy mind, indigestion, body stiffness, or gaining more than 1 kg (2 lb) overnight (inflammatory fluid).

FOODS LEAST LIKELY TO CAUSE INFLAMMATION INCLUDE:
- organic poultry and grass-fed meats
- fish
- seasonal vegetables — except nightshades such as tomatoes, potatoes, capsicums (peppers) and eggplants (aubergines)
- seasonal fruits, and dried fruits without sulfur dioxide
- herbs and spices (except chilli)

- coconut products
- pre-soaked seeds
- natural wholefood sweeteners such as stevia or pure raw honey
- bone broths
- cacao butter
- apple cider vinegar
- herbal teas

These are the rudimentary foods you should base your eating around for 4 weeks as an initial elimination phase before you begin the Supercharge Your Gut two-day maintenance program. This will reset your body to communicate very clearly to you when foods are causing you problems. Keep a food diary and take close note of any physical symptoms that may point to a potential trigger food.

After an initial 6 weeks of basic eating, you may have identified how certain foods cause inflammation. You can then, one by one, every two days, reintroduce the least inflammatory foods, working up to the more likely trigger foods, to see what your body tells you.

These foods include different types of nuts, dairy (beginning with ghee, then butter, yoghurt or kefir, cheese then finally milk), eggs, grains (beginning with gluten-free grains, moving on to gluten-containing grains), lentils and beans, and nightshade vegetables, such as tomatoes and potatoes.

Document in your food diary the inflammatory impact these newly reintroduced foods have on your body.

When you're testing out particular foods, bear in mind that it's quite common to react to foods from the same group, such as nightshades, legumes, starches, crucifers, citrus and FODMAPs.

If you notice an inflammatory food, remove it from your diet for a week, reintroduce it and note your response again. This will make it very clear what isn't serving your body. When you're reintroducing foods, try to have a positive mindset, and not be too anxious about it. Your body should be in a relaxed state to stimulate the process of digestion.

Make this part of a lifestyle approach that you revisit and revise every few months to keep the gut-loving flowing — and remember, diversity is key, so aim not to eat the same foods every day, increase the amount of different types of foods you eat, and rotate your reintroductions.

You're an individual, so you don't need to follow a cookie-cutter approach when it comes to your diet — just give yourself permission to love the process.

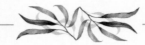

FIVE GREAT INGREDIENTS TO SUPPORT THE GUT LINING

When restoring your digestive tract, you can support the process with nourishing foods that contain key nutrients to promote the repair of the intestinal walls and the growth of good flora within them. Try adding these go-to foods to your gut-friendly shopping cart.

If you're new to them, start small by adding one or two of these ingredients to your meals each week, or having a cup of bone broth on your Supercharged Gut days.

1 BONE BROTHS

Soothing, immune-boosting, anti-inflammatory and nutrient-dense, bone broths offer a huge array of easily absorbable minerals, such as calcium, magnesium, phosphorus, silicon, sulfur and trace minerals, and help heal and seal the digestive tract. You'll find a range of bone broth recipes on pages 192–198.

2 GELATINE

Gelatine works wonders on the gut lining by sealing damage caused by lifestyle factors such as poor diet and stress, and repairing the effects of leaky gut. It can also improve digestive strength by enhancing secretion of gastric acids that help break down food (including dairy in intolerant individuals), making it easier to absorb nutrients in the small intestine. Gelatine also absorbs water, which helps keep fluid in the digestive tract, promoting good intestinal transit and healthy bowel movements.

Apart from consuming it in very jelly-like bone broths, you can also buy dehydrated gelatine to use in jellies and desserts, or add to smoothies and soups. Ensure the product is 100 per cent natural, and if possible from pasture-raised, ethically treated cows.

3 ALOE VERA

Aloe vera leaf is high in vitamins and minerals, and has anti-inflammatory properties that help relax the intestinal tract and heal any damage. It contains enzymes that help break down food, promoting regular bowel movements, and acts as a prebiotic to help feed the good bacteria in your gut. You can buy aloe vera in liquid form, and add it to desserts and smoothies.

4 SLIPPERY ELM

Long used by indigenous cultures, this South American herb comes from the inner bark of the elm tree. It is widely known as a digestive aid, and works by forming a soothing film over the mucous membranes it comes into contact with, relieving digestive pain and inflammation, making it particularly helpful in colitis and irritable bowel syndrome. Slippery elm contains a fibre that forms a gel or mucilage, which acts as a lubricant throughout the stomach and small and large intestines.

To protect your gut lining from inflammation, add a teaspoon of slippery elm to a glass of water and drink half an hour before meals.

Slippery elm is also wonderful for easing diarrhoea and constipation. Add 1–2 tablespoons to a smoothie or your morning porridge.

5 TURMERIC

Turmeric is a powerful anti-inflammatory that will help soothe the gut and alleviate congestion. It improves digestion and reduces gas and bloating by increasing production of the enzymes that break down fat, protein and carbohydrates. Turmeric's antibacterial properties also help rid the digestive system of harmful bacteria, giving the helpful bacteria a chance to flourish. It can be added to soups, smoothies, herb teas and curries. Use a bioactive type, or with a pinch of black pepper to increase absorption, or heat with coconut milk to release curcumin, its active anti-inflammatory ingredient.

THE IMPORTANCE OF FIBRE

Fibre is of paramount importance to the health of your gut and digestive system. Fibres are non-digestible carbohydrates from plant sources, and getting the right kinds in your diet will give you the best chance of creating a healthy community of gut bacteria and smooth digestion. Fibre can be soluble or insoluble.

- SOLUBLE FIBRE: Dissolves in water, and is slower to digest as it attracts water to form a gel. Types include oatmeal, psyllium husks, acacia fibres, berries, lentils (soaked for easier digestion), fruit and vegetables.
- INSOLUBLE FIBRE: Doesn't dissolve in water. It passes through the digestive system relatively intact and speeds up the passage of food waste through your gut. Sources include grains, nuts, seeds, beans, fruit and vegetables.

While insoluble fibres are great for flushing out pollutants from the body, an excess of these fibres can be irritating. Too much roughage can also bind to minerals such as zinc, magnesium, calcium and iron, preventing their absorption.

Soluble fibres, on the other hand, are the ones you really should focus on for improved gut health. When you eat the soluble fibres found in whole plant foods, your gut bacteria ferment them into short-chain fatty acids such as butyrate, propionate and acetate, which nourish your gut. This is wonderful for maintaining the integrity of your gut lining, improving digestion, increasing the absorption of minerals and even assisting immune system function.

HEALTHY SOURCES OF SOLUBLE FIBRE INCLUDE:

- sweet potatoes, carrots and root vegetables
- green leafy vegetables
- berries
- nuts and seeds (pre-soaked to make digestion easier)

PREBIOTICS AND PROBIOTICS: WHAT'S THE DIFFERENCE?

They sound virtually the same, but prebiotics and probiotics have very different functions inside our digestive systems.

Each of us can carry up to 2 kg (4½ lb) of microbes in our gut. It can seem unfathomable at times to comprehend that we aren't alone in our inner universe, and that our bodies are dependent on a harmonious partnership with the complex ecosystem than lives within us.

We know that our microbiome is the community of bacteria that resides within our body and is responsible for more than just our digestive health. Within our gut, a healthy microflora involves a greater number of probiotic (or friendly) bacteria, and a smaller amount of pathogenic bacteria. However, our friendly bugs need to be fed to maintain the survival and proliferation of their colony; due to the popularity of paleo and keto-style diets, many prebiotic-rich foods are being overlooked, and this can be detrimental to gut health.

This is where prebiotics come in — and in simple terms, they act as a food for our good bacteria, as they're high in special types of fibre.

Probiotic and fermented foods have been getting a lot of attention of late — but it's prebiotics that do all the behind-the-scenes work in our tummies. Without them, probiotic bugs have a poor chance of surviving. While probiotics are live organisms, prebiotics are the components of our food that are otherwise not easily digested, but are thoroughly enjoyed by our beneficial bacteria. These include oligosaccharides such as oligofructose and inulin, which leave behind carbohydrate molecules that are a tasty meal for our microbiome.

Good vegetable sources of prebiotics include fresh dandelion greens, Jerusalem artichokes, onions, leeks, chives, garlic, endive, asparagus, radicchio, chicory, shallots, spring onions (scallions), beetroot (beet), fennel bulbs, green peas, snow peas (mangetout) and savoy cabbage.

Prebiotic fruits with extra punch include avocados, custard apples, nectarines, white peaches, persimmons, bananas, apples, pomegranates and figs.

I encourage you to incorporate some of these delicious prebiotic foods into your diet. Because once you've established the good gut bugs, to help them flourish and give them a stable home you've got to feed them!

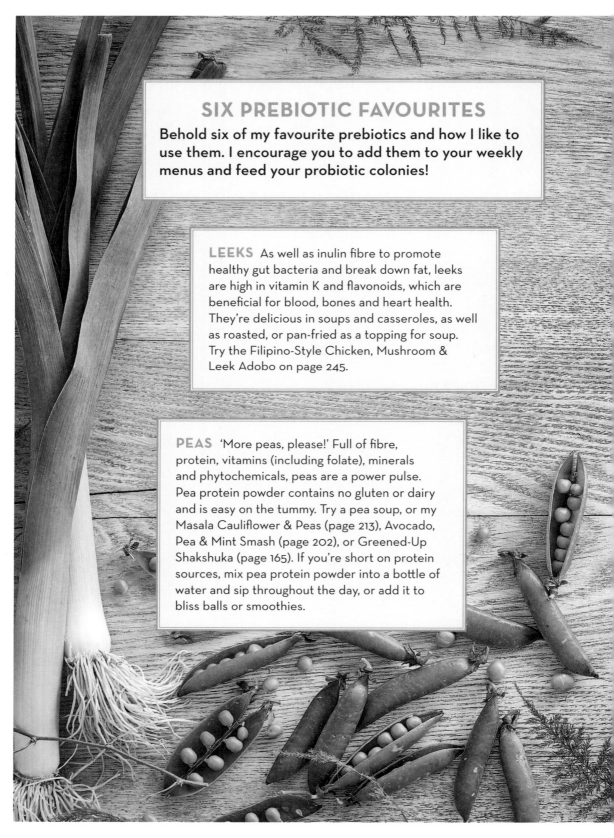

SIX PREBIOTIC FAVOURITES

Behold six of my favourite prebiotics and how I like to use them. I encourage you to add them to your weekly menus and feed your probiotic colonies!

LEEKS As well as inulin fibre to promote healthy gut bacteria and break down fat, leeks are high in vitamin K and flavonoids, which are beneficial for blood, bones and heart health. They're delicious in soups and casseroles, as well as roasted, or pan-fried as a topping for soup. Try the Filipino-Style Chicken, Mushroom & Leek Adobo on page 245.

PEAS 'More peas, please!' Full of fibre, protein, vitamins (including folate), minerals and phytochemicals, peas are a power pulse. Pea protein powder contains no gluten or dairy and is easy on the tummy. Try a pea soup, or my Masala Cauliflower & Peas (page 213), Avocado, Pea & Mint Smash (page 202), or Greened-Up Shakshuka (page 165). If you're short on protein sources, mix pea protein powder into a bottle of water and sip throughout the day, or add it to bliss balls or smoothies.

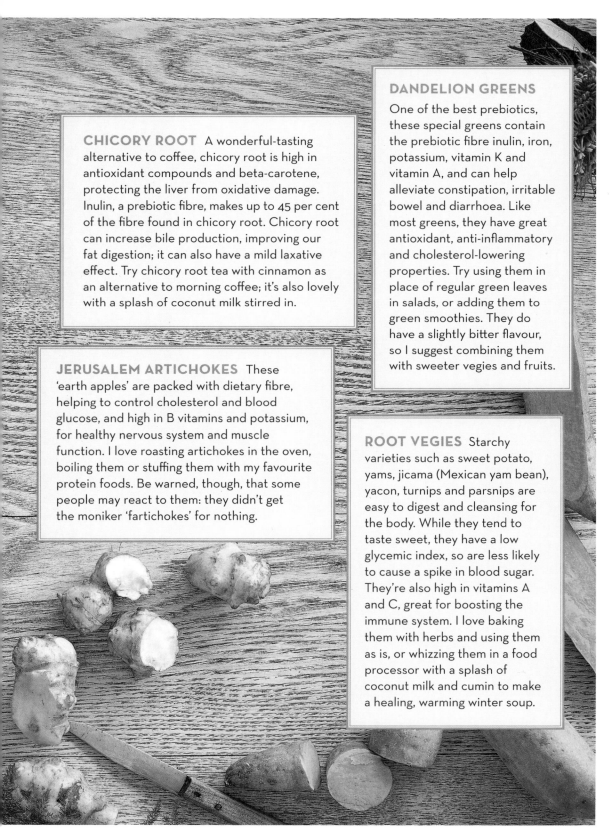

CHICORY ROOT A wonderful-tasting alternative to coffee, chicory root is high in antioxidant compounds and beta-carotene, protecting the liver from oxidative damage. Inulin, a prebiotic fibre, makes up to 45 per cent of the fibre found in chicory root. Chicory root can increase bile production, improving our fat digestion; it can also have a mild laxative effect. Try chicory root tea with cinnamon as an alternative to morning coffee; it's also lovely with a splash of coconut milk stirred in.

DANDELION GREENS
One of the best prebiotics, these special greens contain the prebiotic fibre inulin, iron, potassium, vitamin K and vitamin A, and can help alleviate constipation, irritable bowel and diarrhoea. Like most greens, they have great antioxidant, anti-inflammatory and cholesterol-lowering properties. Try using them in place of regular green leaves in salads, or adding them to green smoothies. They do have a slightly bitter flavour, so I suggest combining them with sweeter vegies and fruits.

JERUSALEM ARTICHOKES These 'earth apples' are packed with dietary fibre, helping to control cholesterol and blood glucose, and high in B vitamins and potassium, for healthy nervous system and muscle function. I love roasting artichokes in the oven, boiling them or stuffing them with my favourite protein foods. Be warned, though, that some people may react to them: they didn't get the moniker 'fartichokes' for nothing.

ROOT VEGIES Starchy varieties such as sweet potato, yams, jicama (Mexican yam bean), yacon, turnips and parsnips are easy to digest and cleansing for the body. While they tend to taste sweet, they have a low glycemic index, so are less likely to cause a spike in blood sugar. They're also high in vitamins A and C, great for boosting the immune system. I love baking them with herbs and using them as is, or whizzing them in a food processor with a splash of coconut milk and cumin to make a healing, warming winter soup.

RESISTANT STARCH: FRIEND OR FOE?

Just like teeny-weeny microscopic babies with wide open mouths, your gut microbes await your feeding, and just like humans, they can be fed junk, or nourished with the foods they evolved to thrive on — prebiotics, those special carbohydrate molecules that survive our digestive tract and reach our colon intact before selectively feeding specific strains of bacteria.

Resistant starch is another prebiotic that reaches the colon, having 'resisted' digestion. There are different four types of resistant starch.

- RS TYPE 1: Found in grains, seeds and legumes, where the fibre is bound up in the fibrous cell walls of the plants.
- RS TYPE 2: Found in potatoes, green bananas and plantains, this is starch with a high amylose content, which is indigestible in its raw state; when cooked, the resistant starch is removed and the food becomes digestible to us. Plantain flour and green banana flour can be added to smoothies (15–30 g/ ^{1}/2–1 oz daily).
- RS TYPE 3: This forms when type 1 or type 2 resistant starches are cooked, then cooled to below 54°C (130°F). Heating these foods back up to high temperatures will again convert the starch into the digestible form, where it will not last to feed the bacteria in the colon. Examples include lentils, potato and rice that have been cooked and cooled.
- RS TYPE 4: This is the synthetic form of resistant starch, including Hi-maize resistant starch, which has been chemically modified and which I would personally not recommend. It is being increasingly used in commercial breads, pasta and snack bars.

The first three types of resistant starch are your friends, and will help feed your good microbes so they produce short-chain fatty acids, the most significant of which are acetate, butyrate and propionate. Butyrate is of special importance due to its beneficial effects on the colon and overall health — it enters the bloodstream through the colon, having an anti-inflammatory effect on the body, as well as decreasing intestinal permeability and the effects of leaky gut.

REPLENISHING YOUR MICROBIOME

Our 'germophobic' lifestyle of antibacterial room sprays, cleaning and personal care products, chlorinated water and antibiotics can also take a toll on our microbiome.

To replenish your strains of good bacteria, try to consume small amounts of probiotic-rich foods at least a few times each week. I like to take a probiotic supplement daily, and consume a range of fermented and probiotic foods to widen the diversity of my good bacteria, as different strains have different health benefits, ranging from increased serotonin production to an improved metabolism. I use these probiotics as an insurance policy, rotating them each month or two to ensure a broader spectrum of probiotic strains.

Some sensitive tummies can suffer from gas and bloating when probiotic-rich foods are first implemented. It's best to start slowly with a teaspoon a day and build up from there.

I've listed my favourite probiotic-rich foods and their benefits below. Other good sources include yoghurt or coconut yoghurt, coconut water kefir or water kefir, kombucha, miso paste and natto (a Japanese fermented soybean product).

Incorporating a range of the following ingredients into your soups, smoothies, bakes and slow-cooked dishes will help contribute to a thriving inner ecosystem that will benefit the wellbeing of your entire body.

But remember, baby steps.

SAUERKRAUT

Sauerkraut is finely cut cabbage that has been through a fermentation process, making it far more nutritious than the raw variety. It dates back to the Ancient Romans, who took it with them on long journeys. As well as improving digestive health, sauerkraut contains high levels of iron, which is good for boosting energy and preventing anaemia. However, it can be high in sodium, so be wary when choosing store-bought varieties. I like adding sauerkraut to my eggs in the morning, on top of my warmed vegie bowls, and alongside hearty stews.

KEFIR

Similar to a drinkable yoghurt, kefir is a thick, creamy, nutrient-dense fermented milk product, rich in vitamin B12, calcium, magnesium, vitamin K2, biotin and folate. It can support the immune system, increase bone density, enhance detoxification and help with digestive issues. It's made using kefir grains — little structures that act as homes to the live bacteria and yeast cultures. You can drink kefir straight up, add it to smoothies, whip it up like cream cheese or use it instead of yoghurt in a dressing.

MICROALGAE

You may have heard of 'superfood' green powders that include wacky-sounding ingredients such as chlorella and spirulina, but what you may not know is that these foods can act as powerful probiotics. Green powders are made of different nutrient-dense organisms found in salt water. Spirulina is comprised of more than 70 per cent protein, as well as vitamin E, chlorophyll and fatty acids. Chlorella is a green microalga filled with chlorophyll, protein and carotenoids. Chlorophyll, found in both spirulina and chlorella, is a powerful probiotic in the gut. You can mix these powders into a glass of water, or add them to green smoothies.

KIMCHI

Kimchi is a traditional Korean food created by fermenting vegetables, especially cabbage, with seasonings such as chilli, garlic, turmeric and ginger. This antioxidant mix contains bacteria to help the gastrointestinal and immune systems. Kimchi is high in enzymes, making it great for digestion, with an added kick from the seasoning spices. You can use it as a condiment, but add it sparingly as it can be spicy hot.

PICKLES

Here we're talking about pickles that have been lacto-fermented (i.e. fermented in salty water, not vinegar), making them rich in probiotics and full of live bacteria. Pickles are best when they're organic and, if possible, locally made. Add them to sandwiches or toss through salads for a salty probiotic kick. Or try the Turmeric Pickled Eggs on page 168.

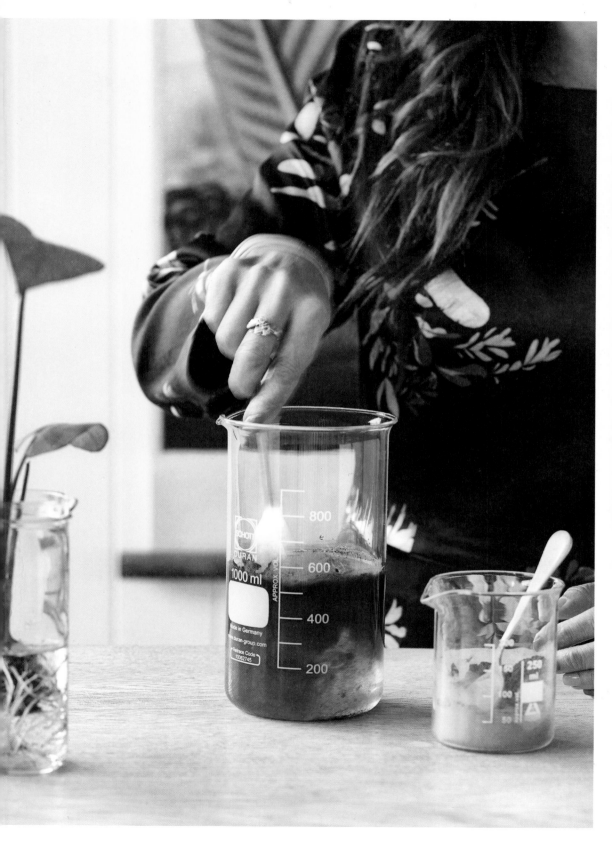

DO I NEED DIGESTIVE ENZYMES?

Digestive enzymes are another vital piece of the gut-health puzzle. They break down larger molecules of food into more easily absorbed particles, and so are essential for good digestion and nutrient absorption. Without digestive enzymes we cannot process our food.

Through a range of complicated processes, digestive enzymes break down food into amino acids, fatty acids, cholesterol, simple sugars and nucleic acids, whereas intestinal enzymes metabolise sugars, and pancreatic enzymes deal with fats and amino acids.

Digestive enzymes help to heal leaky gut by taking stress off the gastrointestinal tract, they assist the body to digest gluten and lactose, and help to counteract the enzyme inhibitors and anti-nutrients found in nuts, seeds, beans, potatoes and lentils.

People who have age-related enzyme insufficiency, leaky gut, liver disease, Crohn's disease and other digestive diseases may require digestive enzymes in the form of supplements. However, certain foods can naturally enhance digestive enzyme production, so if you feel like you need a little help, put these in your kitchen medicine cupboard.

- PINEAPPLE: Contains the enzyme bromelain, which can aid in the digestion of proteins.
- MANGO: Contains enzymes such as mangiferin, katechol oxidase and lactase, which can all help with metabolising sugars and proteins.
- PAPAYA: Contains the digestive enzyme papain, which is most concentrated in the fruit when it is unripe. Papain is wonderful for helping to digest tough meat fibres, breaking them down into smaller proteins, peptides (short chains of and amino acids.
- OLIVE OIL AND LEMON: In combination, these are great for digestion. Olive oil triggers the release of a hormone that improves fat and protein digestion, and lemon juice helps get your saliva flowing, speeding up the digestive process from the beginning. A great way to improve bile flow and digestion is to mix the two ingredients together and take each morning or on an empty stomach. Try the Olive Oil & Lemon Shot on page 146.

- FENUGREEK: Traditionally used to aid digestion and maintain a healthy appetite. Studies have found it to help suppress increases in blood glucose and is highly anti-inflammatory to the gut.[24] The Fenugreek Pre-Digestive Tea on page 146 acts as a decongestant to the bile ducts and supports normal bile flow.
- CINNAMON: Wonderful for increasing bile flow, and promoting healthy glucose metabolism by stimulating the natural production of insulin.

Another way you can help support the digestive process and assist nutrient uptake is by eating foods that promote the flow of bile.

Bile movers, or cholagogues, work by stimulating bile from the liver through to the gallbladder and then into the intestines, ensuring the optimum breakdown and uptake of nutrients.

The secretion of bile is of great help to the whole digestive and assimilative process. It promotes fat digestion, and helps the flow of digestive enzymes through the pancreas and the transport of vital fat-soluble vitamins and fatty acids. It also acts as a natural cleansing laxative, scrubbing the digestive villi lining the small intestine, detoxifying wastes and removing bad cholesterol from the body.

Try these natural cholagogue ingredients.

- TURMERIC: Has an anti-inflammatory effect on the gut and helps improve bile flow.
- BITTER LEAFY GREENS AND HERBS: Chicory, rosemary, rocket (arugula), kale, nettles, turnip greens and watercress are all wonderful at switching on digestive enzyme production and salivary glands. The cellulose in the greens also helps to remove bile toxins from the body.
- GLOBE ARTICHOKE: Has wonderful bile-enhancing capabilities through stimulating the gallbladder. It also contains a substance called cinarin, which is beautiful for detoxifying the liver.
- CELERY: Contains unique compounds in which sodium is bonded with many bioactive trace minerals and nutrients. Celery juice in the morning is a nifty way to strengthen your digestion for the day, and over time, the minerals and mineral salts will help to restore your stomach's natural hydrochloric acid.

Try including more sources of all these foods to increase your natural digestive enzyme production and support a healthy well-loved gut.

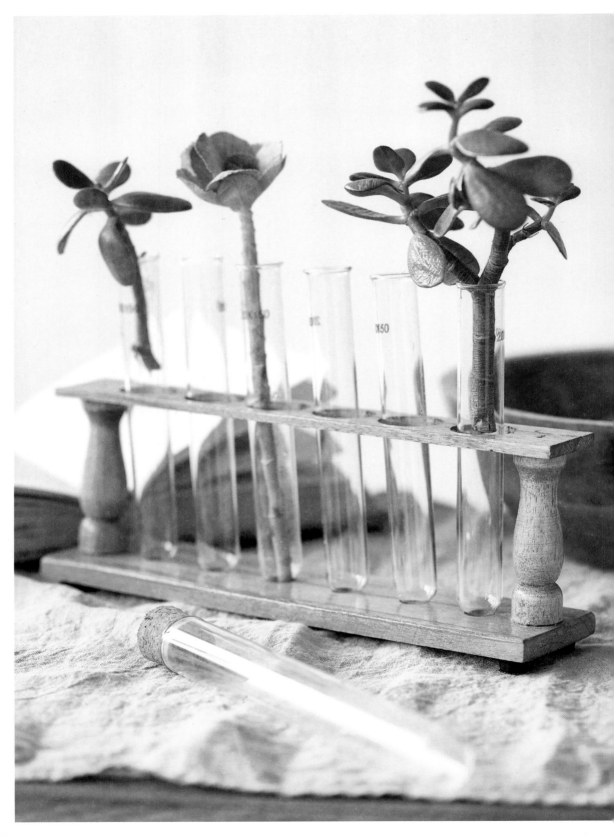

THE BALANCED GUT

It's about time you gave your hardworking gut a round of applause. Because it's been the cornerstone to your health up until now, it deserves a chance to get back on its feet, have time to rest and flourish within a stable environment.

Help get your gut back on an even keel by adopting practices to balance your contrasting nervous system centres, and embracing the art of eating consciously.

BEING BEHIND THE WHEEL

Knowing what to feed the gut for ideal digestion is all well and good, but how do you incorporate a new plan of gut-supporting action in a simple and balanced way?

To truly supercharge your gut, you need to have a fresh and open mindset. Many people outsource the primary responsibility for their health to doctors, diet books or the advice of the food pyramid. However, this may never produce the level of vitality you truly desire, because no health expert or program will ever be able to cater for your every unique, individual needs the way you can.

While it's valuable to seek professional guidance and lean on the research of specialists and scientists, you alone are the daily steward of your body, who makes the everyday choices affecting your larger future. You're the one behind the steering wheel on your own health journey. Tune in to your body and your thoughts, and steer yourself in a way that's appropriate for your individual path.

As you get behind the wheel on the road towards gut healing and maintenance, you'll find that there'll be times to put your foot on the accelerator, and times to shift right down to first gear and move much more slowly.

Only you will know intuitively when the time is right to take the full-speed-ahead approach. You'll feel ready for it. These times will involve fuelling yourself with healing foods that boost your metabolism and detoxification, adding more fire to your digestion, and ramping up physical movement.

You'll also definitely know when to pull back, slow riiigghhhht down and shift the gears towards self-care, mindfulness, and gentler gut-soothing recipes for broths and simple soups that are easily digested.

These times are just as important on your journey to better health, and act as a convalescence for your digestive system. You'll notice after these restorative, slow times of healing, your energy will gradually increase and you'll be ready to ramp up into fifth gear again.

Wherever you're at, listen to your body, and adjust your speed and approach accordingly.

The fast and the slow steering stages might seem contradictory, but they actually complement one another. This is very similar to the way your autonomic nervous system works.

Within your autonomic nervous system, you have both your sympathetic and your parasympathetic nervous systems working to control your entire body. These are the competing systems that let you speed up or slow down — to 'fight or take flight', or 'rest and digest'.

These contrasting nervous systems are essential for our survival. And a balance between the two is vital for the rest, healing and active repair needed to have your gut working to its full potential.

THE STRESS RESPONSE

Let's delve a little deeper into our sympathetic nervous system. We all know that high stress isn't good for us, but it's actually the low-level ongoing stress — known as chronic stress — that can wreak havoc on our gut.

When we think of stress, many of us think of being pressured by bosses at work, not having enough time to do all the things we need to do, or juggling too many family, social or work commitments.

But over-exercising, not getting enough sleep and not feeling moments of joy and pleasure in our daily life can also cause stress that affects our gut.

Stress produces too much cortisol in our bodies, and it's cortisol that activates our sympathetic nervous system, which is linked to the 'flight or fight' response. When the sympathetic nervous system is activated, the parasympathetic nervous system that controls our 'rest and digest' mode must be suppressed, since they cannot operate simultaneously.

Usually when we're eating, the parasympathetic nervous system is at play. This is important because for the body to best use food energy, the enzymes and hormones controlling digestion and absorption must be working.

When you have a stressed-out, cortisol-flooded body, digestion and nutrient absorption are compromised, and the mucosal lining can become irritated and inflamed. Mucosal inflammation can in turn lead to the increased production of cortisol, creating a vicious cycle. Stress-induced changes to the gut include alterations to gastric secretions, gut motility, mucosal permeability, barrier function (leading to leaky gut) and increased sensitivity.[25]

The first step to controlling stress is to be mindful of how big a role it's playing in our lives, start noticing when it affects us and what triggers it — then be prepared to hit the snooze button.

The next step is to look at simple ways of minimising stress. If you're always stressed about being late to work, perhaps you could start getting ready a little earlier, or prepare what you need the night before.

It seems obvious, but these simple steps can make a very big impact in reducing stress levels and aiding overall health.

APPLYING THE BREAKS

When you need to put the gears into reverse, gentle exercise and meditation can help. Regular exercise is a major player when it comes to combating stress.

So what types of exercises are best?

It's good to remember that when you exercise you're putting your body under a form of stress that it will need to recover from. So while caring for your gut, it's best to keep exercise nice and simple.

If exercise is something you haven't done for a long time, ease into it and take it slowly. Start off with short 15–20 minute walks daily and work your way up to longer ones. While walking, concentrate on deep breathing and relaxation, enjoy the fresh air and really unwind.

YOGA

Yoga is perfect for supporting and healing the gut, as many of the breathing and postural practices are directly aimed at the digestive tract (see page 95). Your yoga routine doesn't need to be complex; a basic restorative yoga practice can improve your body's ability to digest and detoxify, as well as improve your mood, motivation and energy levels. Certain yoga postures aim to massage your internal organs, and alternatively constrict and stimulate the flow of blood to specific areas of the body, maximising the absorption of nutrients and assisting the elimination process. Yoga can also help with symptoms such as bloating and constipation.

MEDITATION

Meditation can be used as a tool to reset our 'rest and digest' relaxation response.

As a yoga and meditation teacher, I want to share some simple ways to take your foot off the pedal and ease into cruise control.

- BREATHING: Voluntary movement of the organs inside your body helps send signals to your brain that all is existing in peace and harmony. Practising some deep, even breathing throughout the day will help make the communication between your brain and your gut smooth and uninterrupted.
- NOTICING YOUR POSTURE: Stress doesn't only mean an emotional, mental state of discomfort, but also the physical stress on your joints and muscles. Stretching out a tight muscle, correcting an awkward position, relieving a tightened chest and so on can send life-changing messages throughout your body. Lengthening your torso will create digestive space to reduce bloating and gut discomfort, thus promoting an anti-inflammatory response accompanied by the 'rest and digest' response.
- MINDFULNESS AND RELAXATION: I love that mindfulness is actually classified as a form of relaxation. Just being aware of your surroundings, appreciating every movement, every mouthful, every colour and every person will assist in your quest to reset your body's 'rest and digest' mode.

THE SLOW FOOD MOVEMENT

When you look around, fast food is everywhere, with new fast-food chains popping up on every street corner and people chomping through their food faster than Usain Bolt approaching the finishing line.

Living in our fast-paced world, we expect everything to occur quickly — from the food that we order to the pace at which we devour it. Quality has been replaced by quantity, and a lot of it. This is part of a wider phenomenon known as 'McDonaldization', where we can be in any city in the world and receive exactly the same burger, cola and fries as we would at home. Homogenisation on a global scale.

It's time to start thinking of food as care fuel. Real food is like premium petrol; fast food is like filling our tank up with cheap gas and expecting our engine to run just as well. Highly processed fast food is high in calories, refined carbohydrates, added sugars, unhealthy fats and extreme salt levels. The only thing it's not high in is nutrients. And it's not good for our good gut bacteria, or gut diversity.

To give our digestive system time and space to digest, I'm calling for a new slow food revolution.

Welcome to the Slow Food movement. If you're not familiar with it, Slow Food arose as a grassroots movement in 1989 to counteract the rise of McDonaldization and cheap, unhealthy fast food, and to help preserve local culinary traditions around the world. It invites us to slow down and reconnect with food, and savour the pleasures of eating real food — to enjoy quality ingredients, grown and produced locally, in an environmentally sustainable way.

Slow foods are good for the soul. Not only do they taste delicious, they have the power to improve our digestion and gut health.

The first stage of digestion occurs before food is even placed in our mouth. The smell and thought of food wakes up and excites our salivary glands in anticipation of a meal — you know the feeling when a batch of muffins comes out of the oven, or you feast your eyes on a slow-cooked meal? This lets the stomach and brain know that food is going to arrive, and triggers the production of our stomach and digestive juices. Only when these juices and enzymes are produced can the stomach be in a position to break down the food we're about to eat.

Our olfactory nerves contribute to the sensation of taste by picking up the aroma of the food and passing the sensation of smell to the brain. Looking, tasting and smelling food stimulates the salivary glands, and an enzyme in the saliva called amylase begins the breakdown of carbohydrates (starch) into simple sugars, such as maltose. Amylase is also secreted by the pancreas.

Consuming our food slowly and mindfully prepares our body to digest its contents much better and absorb nutrients properly. When we eat too quickly, our body reacts negatively, with symptoms such as heartburn, burping, gas and indigestion.

For our gut to function at its peak, one thing is evident: 'slow and steady wins the race'.

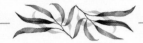

EATING CONSCIOUSLY

So how do you incorporate the Slow Food principles at home while still keeping up with day-to-day life? These simple tips will steer you back into the slow lane.

EAT CONSCIOUSLY: You don't need to chew every mouthful 20 times — food is something that should be enjoyed, and should never be a burden. I do, however, suggest chewing foods slowly. Making time if you can to sit down to a delicious meal and eat it slowly keeps you more in line with your body processes. You'll have less chance of overeating if you experience the feeling of getting full.

PUT DOWN UTENSILS BETWEEN BITES: This can help with slowing down how quickly you're eating. It gives you time to chew your food before mindlessly taking in another mouthful.

FORGET THE FAST-FOOD MANTRA: Good things do take time. Quality food can take more time to prepare than picking up or ordering in a fast-food alternative, but it's worth enjoying and appreciating it for the taste and health benefits alone, especially when you can also enjoy the smells, flavours, colours, textures and even the very process of making your own food.

TURN THE TELLY OFF! When the screen is on, it's easy to gulp and gulp and gulp. Sitting down at a table instead of being mesmerised by a computer screen or television can help us eat more mindfully and find our sweet digestive spot.

It's time to set a new pace, for gutness sake, and slow down both the food we're eating and the way we're eating it. It's time to start chewing to a new rhythm. Let's eat consciously and move away from the 'McDonaldization' of food, back to a more natural and enjoyable way of life.

TUMMY-LOVING PRACTICAL TIPS

Vagus nerve push-ups? Yes they're a thing! Stay happy and loved-up with my handy tips for nurturing and strengthening your gut–brain axis. Learn how to master their messages and bring about harmonious synergy between both your gut and brain.

MASTERING YOUR NERVOUS SYSTEM

In the tale of two brains, we learnt that the brain and gut are closely connected, and the pathway that links these two completely isolated areas of the body is the vagus nerve. It's a super-important piece of biology for you to wrap your head around if you want a complete picture of the way your moods, energy levels, concentration and mental capacity function.

Your vagus nerve is a mind–body feedback loop, where messages from the gut can travel 'upstream' to your brain. They can also travel 'downstream' from your conscious mind through the vagus nerve (via efferent nerves), signalling your organs to create an inner calm so you can 'rest and digest' during times of safety, or to prepare your body for 'fight or flight' in dangerous situations.

Healthy vagus nerve communication between your gut and your brain will help to slow you down, like the brakes on your car, through neurotransmitters that will lower your heart rate and blood pressure, and help your heart and organs slow down rather than operate via stress-based responses that put further stress on your digestive processes.

Strong evidence from animal studies is showing that pathogenic bacteria and inflammation of the gut can activate the vagus nerve through an anti-inflammatory reflex that can have negative consequences for brain function and mood.

Other studies suggest that distinct microbial and nutritional stimuli in the gut can create corresponding changes in brain neurochemistry, and thereby behaviour.[26] In other words, how you feed and care for your microbiome through your lifestyle choices can either heal or harm your brain and mood function.

Knowing how your digestive system and brain function are connected is incredibly liberating. It empowers you to make simple tweaks in your diet and lifestyle, to help maximise the odds of moving past those health struggles you may have believed have always been part of who you are.

NURTURING YOUR GUT–BRAIN AXIS

If you're looking to take your connection to new heights, here are a few of my favourite tips for strengthening your brain–gut axis and mastering its messages.

- Promote healthy circadian rhythms by getting to bed between 9 pm and 10 pm, and waking naturally with the sun if possible.
- Avoid white and blue sources of light (fluorescent lighting, mobile phones, tablets and TV screens) after the sun goes down.
- Walk or exercise outdoors early in the morning, with the morning sun in your eyes. The angle of the sun will stimulate your brain in a way that promotes positive mood and brain function, through stimulating the pineal gland and melatonin production.
- Use essential oils and aromatherapy. Choose uplifting citrus-based blends during the day to improve mental focus and energy, and lavender oil in the evenings to calm your nervous system after a stressful day.
- Journal your emotions and reflect on them. Before going to sleep, write down 10 things you were grateful for in your day.
- Practise rhythmic forms of exercise regularly, such as swimming, yoga and jogging.
- Practise mindfulness and meditation.
- Reduce your use of stimulants such as caffeine, which can exacerbate 'fight or flight' responses.
- Unplug from technology in the home. Don't sleep with your phone in your room. Yes, that means you! No, you cannot just quickly check Instagram.

Because the vagus nerve is a 'two-way street' of consequences looping from your brain to your gut, embracing a lifestyle that nurtures the health of both camps is necessary for mastering your nervous system so that there's a constant, harmonious synergy operating in this pathway, and both your gut and brain stay happy and loved-up!

The recipes in this book will tackle the gut end of things, but there are other practical steps you can take to help foster a healthy communication between your brain and your gut.

EXERCISES TO STRENGTHEN YOUR VAGUS NERVE

Practise one or two of the following exercises a day to improve the strength of the vagus nerve and gut–brain axis.

- GARGLING: Drink a large glass of water, gargling each sip until you've finished, to contract the muscles in the back of your throat and activate the vagus nerve.
- SING LOUDLY: In the car, in the shower, wherever you can get away with it! This again will activate the vagus nerve and increase oxygen to the brain.
- GAG: This mightn't seem very fun at all, but activating your gag reflex with your toothbrush is like doing push-ups for the vagus nerve! And one, and two ...
- STEPS VISUALISATION: Visualise your vagus nerve from your brain to your gut as a beautiful old spiral staircase. Start at the top of your brain and breathe in and out for three seconds, looking around and observing the colour of each stair, and breathing out any emotions you may feel. Move down each step in this way until you reach your gut. What do you see? How do you feel? Pause at the bottom in your gut and then move back up in the same manner to the top of the brain.

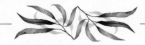

YOGA POSES TO CALM THE BELLY

UTTANASANA (STANDING FORWARD BEND)

1. Start from a standing pose with your big toes touching, heels slightly apart, tailbone tucked under, and arms beside you with your palms facing forwards.
2. Inhale and sweep your arms out to the sides, then up above your head.
3. Exhale and gradually bend forward from your hips, lengthening your spine and lowering your upper body over your legs.
4. Relax your upper body and bring your left hand to your right elbow, and your right hand to your left elbow. (If you feel any discomfort behind your knees or in your hamstrings, feel free to bend your knees.)
5. Hold for 10 breaths, then release slowly, rolling up your spine one vertebra at a time.

PARIPURNA NAVASANA (BOAT POSE)

1. Start in a seated bend position, with your knees pulled up, thighs engaged, and toes pointed towards the ceiling.
2. Keeping your feet together, slowly bring your legs straight up to a 45 degree angle while inhaling, without bending your knees.
3. Without letting the spine collapse, lean back naturally as your legs are raised, so your body looks like a 'V'.
4. Stretch your arms out in front of you at shoulder level.
5. Hold the pose for a count of 8, and then exhale, slowly releasing your arms and legs.

VIPARITA KARANI (LEGS UP THE WALL)

1. Lie on the floor and walk your buttocks towards the wall. Extend your legs straight up the wall. If your hamstrings are tight, walk your hips about 15 cm (6 inches) away from the wall, or bend your knees slightly. Your arms can be out to your sides, palms face-up. Slowly and carefully tuck your chin into your chest, and extend the back of your neck on the floor. Soften your gaze and hold the pose for 2–10 minutes.
2. To come out of the pose, slowly bend your knees and roll over onto your right side, curling up into a foetal position. Linger for a few breaths, then press up until seated.

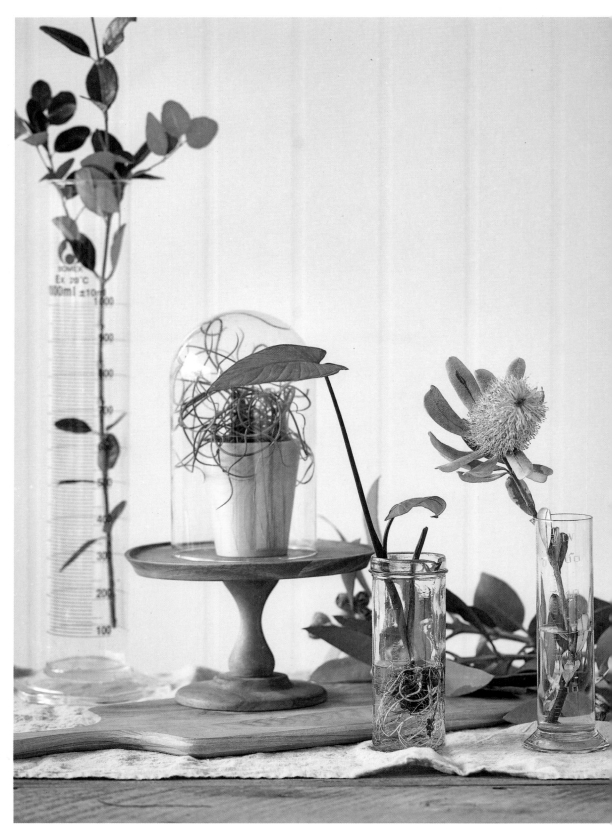

THE SOCIABLE GUT

When learning to care for your gut, or deciding to embark on a maintenance plan for two days a week, don't be too daunted by its social impact on others. Once you employ a few easy organisational skills, you can enjoy fuss-free days and still be able to get friends and family involved. Read on to find out how.

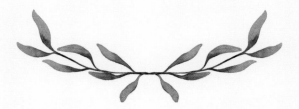

MAKING IT WORK WITH A FAMILY

If you organise yourself, your Supercharged Gut days can be just like any other day — especially if you can encourage a family member to do them with you. On my online gut programs, you'll find many mothers and daughters and sons teaming up. And partners are doing it for themselves too — many of our members are eating the healing soups and finding that kids are also lapping them up.

A great first step is deciding which two days each week you're going to dedicate to maintaining your gut — this will help with forward planning and make for smoother sailing. Try to stick to them to have a routine each week.

- Take 15 minutes on the weekend to map out your week's meals and organise grocery shopping, so there's always something in the house.
- Prepare as many elements as possible in advance over the weekend — for example chop your vegies and place in containers, cook up quinoa, put some spice mixtures together.
- Start by introducing more soups and mash bowls into the family's meals once a week, so that you're all eating the same meal. They could have crusty bread and extra toppings on theirs, such as goat's cheese, pumpkin seeds (pepitas) or coconut flakes.
- If you're cooking a meal for the family — for example chicken with vegetables — why not cook one meal for all of you, then pop your portion into a blender, add some warmed coconut milk and/or stock and turn it into a delicious soup? All you really need to do is make your meals more digestible, so the work is already done for your belly.
- Make extra at dinner time, and blend leftovers for soup or mash bowls to take to work the next day.
- Batch cooking is a great way to get organised. Consider having a batch cooking day, where you freeze your soup into individual portions that can be easily heated up. I generally cook my gut-friendly meals on Sunday afternoon or evening. That way, on my 'on' days, I can just heat and go.
- Make the family overnight smoothie bowls and chia puddings the night before, so you can cruise through the morning rush hour. They can enjoy them with their favourite fruit, yoghurt or toppings.

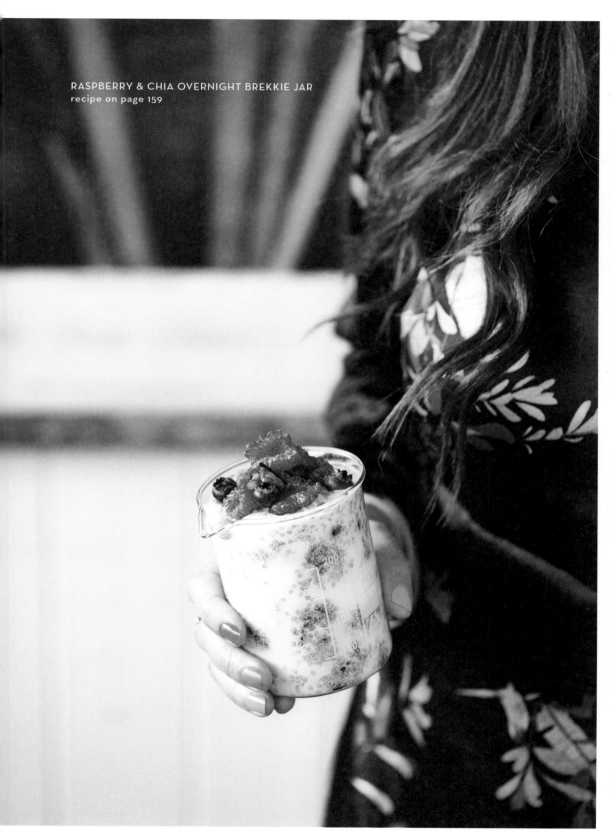

RASPBERRY & CHIA OVERNIGHT BREKKIE JAR
recipe on page 159

- Try introducing smoothies as an after-school snack for your children that you can enjoy too.
- On mornings when you have a bit of time, fire up the slow cooker and make a slow-cooked casserole for the evening, which you can blend into a soup for you if you prefer.

Buying pre-prepared frozen vegies can really help time-poor parents. When I'm in a hurry I look for snap-frozen minted peas and frozen spinach. I use them in soups for myself, but for the family I grab a saucepan, toss the frozen peas straight in, add some feta, grilled bacon and mint or coriander (cilantro), and they really love it.

Also don't forget to prioritise time out for yourself, whether it's having a bath, enjoying a cup of tea or reading a good book — or all three at once! Perhaps organise with your partner in advance to take care of the kids for an hour of 'me' time on your Supercharged Gut evenings.

GETTING BY SOCIALLY

A lot of socialising revolves around food. Whether it's celebrating over dinner or catching up with friends for coffee, food and the topic of food is everywhere.

Changing your eating habits can definitely make social situations quite daunting, or provoke curiosity and even negative responses. Don't worry: it is definitely possible to supercharge your gut and keep your social life at the same time.

The problem with opinions is that everyone has one — your partner, parents, friends, co-workers, and even the shop assistant you barely know. In an ideal world, everyone's opinions would be supportive and informed, but realistically it's easy for us to be negative about things we don't necessarily know much about.

Most of the time the negativity doesn't come at us from a bad place. It's more an automatic response, such as 'Why would you do that?' or 'How do you have the time?' It's not that they purposely want to put you down. Many people feel threatened when they see other people doing something to better themselves or their health. It can be confronting for other people, making them feel bad about things they've been wanting to do but haven't got around to yet — or reminding them of all those things they haven't done, or things they tried in the past that didn't work for them.

It can be helpful to remember this, so it doesn't distract you from the fantastic things you are doing for yourself.

After all is said and done, the most important thing to remember is why? Why are you doing this?

When negativity arises in your life, this is the perfect time to take a moment to reflect. Maybe make a list of the reasons why you've decided to supercharge your gut, and come back to it and read it whenever you're feeling overwhelmed.

Healthy mantras or positive affirmations are fantastic for changing your mindset, especially if doubt is starting to creep in. Short sayings such as 'Nourishing myself is a joyful experience' are perfect to repeat to yourself a few times to get you back into the right headspace. Find one that resonates with you and keep it handy.

Our mind is such a powerful thing, but it can be easily swayed by the opinions of others. Stay on track and remember that so much good is going to come out of this nourishing journey — and that in the end it will all be worth it.

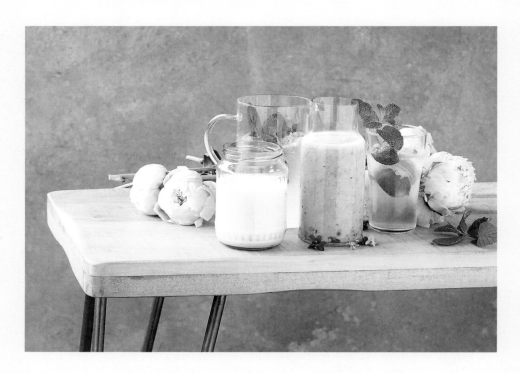

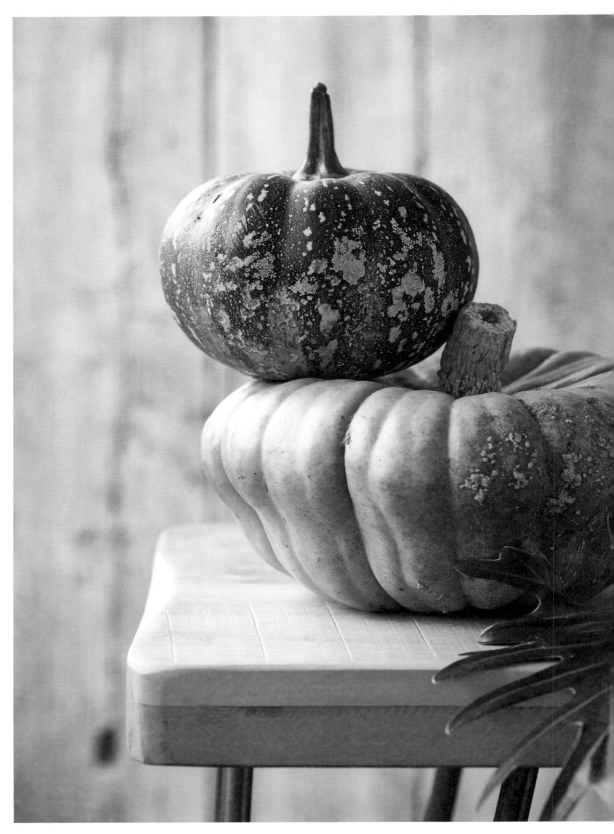

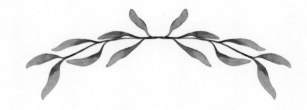

KITCHEN GADGETS
& GUIDES

*Getting down to basics, here are my favourite
kitchen gadgets to make life simple in the kitchen
on your journey to gut health.*

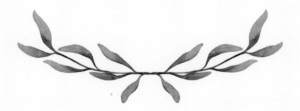

KITCHEN MUST-HAVES

Making easy-to-digest recipes is so simple when you have the right equipment. Having just a few common kitchen items will let you squeeze, blend, brew, whiz, ferment and slow cook your way to better gut health and a happier you.

SLOW COOKER: I've never met a slow cooker I didn't like. Every kitchen should have one of these. Slow cooking is a traditional method of cooking over a gentle flame for a long period of time — but these brilliant appliances make it so easy for you.

The long, slow heating allows the retention of many vitamins and minerals that would otherwise be destroyed by hot, intense heating. Slow cooking gently breaks down the cell walls of vegetables and the fibres in meats, freeing up the nutrients for easy absorption by your digestive system.

This is the perfect device for cooking up a weekly batch of gelatinous, mineral-rich bone broth as a gut-friendly base for all your soups. You can also throw in your soup ingredients in the morning before work, and come home to a deliciously aromatic meal that can also be puréed in the evening if you wish to take the digestibility factor up a notch.

COOKWARE: For creating delicious one-pot soups and stews, I also really love a good ovenproof enamel-coated cast-iron pot with a lid.

These can be purchased relatively inexpensively, and offer a very diffuse, gentle heat compared to the sharp exposure to heat you can get with stainless steel pots. You can sauté, stew, bake and simmer your ingredients away in this kind of pot, either on the stove or in the oven, and you can insert a hand-held stick blender into the pot to purée the contents into easy-to-digest meals.

BLENDER: A blender is vital for some of the recipes in this book, allowing you to quickly whiz up purées, smoothies, nut milks, soups, and thick healthy slurpie desserts in T minus 20 seconds.

If you really want to make the investment, an all-in-one cooker and processor will provide you with a high-speed blender that also cooks, weighs, steams, chops, stirs, mills, kneads and blends virtually anything to the smoothest consistency you could possibly desire.

HAND-HELD STICK BLENDERS: Hand-held blenders (also called immersion or stick blenders) are a very convenient way to purée soups — simply whiz the stick blender around the pot to combine all the ingredients. And afterwards, there's barely anything to clean up — just the handle. Stick blenders are also easy to travel with, if you want to liquefy your meals on the hop.

STORAGE, AND EATING ON THE GO: I'm not a lover of plastic storage. Plastic containers aren't ideal for the environment, and while many claim to be BPA free, I do wonder what other unacknowledged chemicals may be lurking in their structure.

I keep a stash of different glass jars in my cupboard for storing leftover soups, smoothies and slurpie creations, as well as bone broths, nut milks and various other foods. If you leave a couple of inches at the top of your jars, they're also safe for freezing liquids, which can be defrosted by submerging the jar in a sink or large bowl of hot water. You can also freeze portions of smoothie or slurpie desserts in ice cube trays, which can be quickly blended with more liquid for a quick breakfast or evening treat.

When I'm on the go, I pour single-serve portions of smoothies and soups into a glass jar or stainless steel bottle or flask to take with me, so I've always got access to a wholesome snack or meal.

Pyrex storage containers are also handy, as they're made of glass and can double as a cooking vessel in the oven.

MASON JARS: I love mason jars. They come in all shapes and sizes, which makes them very versatile. I use them for storing nut butters, smoothies, seeds, activated nuts, herbs, pickled vegetables, kombucha, and even dinner leftovers for lunch the next day.

You can also use them for instant soups — simply grate up the vegies and greens you're using as your soup base and keep them in a mason jar in the fridge. When the soup craving hits, unscrew the lid, add boiling filtered water and seasonings, and wait 10 minutes. The soup is then ready! How easy is that? And people think being healthy is complicated.

SPIRALISER: You can really pimp up a casserole or soup with some zoodles (zucchini noodles) or spiralised vegetables. Spiralisers are very inexpensive, or you can improvise with a vegetable peeler or mandoline.

BUILDING A HEALTHY SOUP, SMOOTHIE OR SLURPIE

Introducing my five magical steps to get the most out of deliciously digestible meals. It's simple once you learn how.

1 Choose your texture and taste.
2 Create a flavour base.
3 Add the ingredients.
4 Purée.
5 Finish.

FOR A SOUP

1 Choose your desired texture and taste. Do you want your soup to be extra smooth, or have some 'bits' in it? Will you base your soup on water, bone or vegetable broth, or a creamier base like nut milk or coconut cream?

2 Select your ingredients according to the flavour you wish to create. Going for a classic vegetable soup? Base your soup around sautéed onions and garlic, seasonal vegetables and herbs, and your chosen stock or liquid. For a Moroccan kick, combine your meat or vegetables with spices like cumin, coriander and paprika. Other flavour bases could include seasonal greens, or Asian, Indian or Japanese flavours.

3 Sauté your onions or garlic in ghee, coconut or olive oil, add your herbs and dried spices, brown your meats if using, add your chopped vegetables, cover with your chosen liquid and any other liquid flavours like apple cider vinegar, liquid aminos or tamari. Simmer until cooked.

4 Purée with a hand-held stick blender, or in a standing blender, until you achieve your desired consistency.

5 Finish by seasoning with salt and pepper, or some lemon or lime juice for fresh acidity, and maybe some stevia, raw honey or rice malt syrup for sweetness. Serve topped with a swirl of coconut cream, if you like, sprinkled with your choice of extra spices, nutritional yeast, crushed activated nuts or seeds, or freshly chopped herbs.

FOR A SMOOTHIE

1 Do you want a super-smooth smoothie, or would you like to 'chew' it a little? For watery smoothies, opt for coconut water or water as the base. For creamier smoothies, add an avocado or frozen banana, or use nut milks or coconut milk as the base. For thicker smoothies, add chunks of frozen fruit and ice cubes. Soaked chia seeds are also a wonderful thickening agent for smoothies.

2 How do you want to flavour the smoothie? Do you want it to be a berry smoothie, or based around one or several seasonal fruits? For a green smoothie, add vegetables like cucumber, zucchini (courgette), celery and baby spinach. If you need extra sweetness, add a touch of raw honey, rice malt syrup or stevia, or a squeeze of lemon or lime juice for a fresh twist of sourness. For added health benefits you can add in fats like extra virgin coconut oil, flaxseed (linseed) oil, flaxseeds (linseeds) or soaked nuts and seeds, or even probiotics. For a chocolate-flavoured smoothie, add raw cacao powder.

3 Chop any hard ingredients into rough cubes. Add the ingredients to the blender and cover with your chosen liquid (not too much — you can always thin it as you go). If your smoothie doesn't contain frozen fruit, adding around 6 ice cubes will make it much more palatable.

4 Whiz in a blender for around 30 seconds for a more textured smoothie, or about 1 minute for a super-smooth smoothie.

5 Serve topped with sprinkles like chia seeds, cinnamon, and a swirl of coconut cream.

SLURPIES

Slurpies are like an extra-thick smoothie, almost the same texture as Nicecream (see pages 282–286), but served in a tall glass. You can either follow the smoothie guidelines above to build your slurpie, or you can make a smoothie, freeze it in ice cube trays, and use the cubes with a tiny bit of coconut cream or coconut water to get the cubes moving through the blender.

When blending, you may need to stop and help it along a few times with a spatula before it combines into a creamy dreamy slurpie.

My favourite slurpies are based on coconut cream, avocado and frozen banana, as they give the creamiest, thickest texture.

Try the Raspberry & Coconut Yoghurt Slurpie on page 155, then make your own versions of deliciousness.

BEST-EVER BONE BROTHS

Free of genetically modified ingredients, processed salt and the additives found in commercial varieties, homemade bone broths provide an abundance of nutrients and health benefits, while also being simple and economical to prepare.

A meal in themselves, bone broths are so easy to include in everyday recipes, adding wonderful flavour and an extra healing boost to soups, casseroles, curries and tagines, or even when cooking rice or quinoa.

To make the best-ever bone broths, here's all you need to do.

1 SELECT YOUR BONES

- You can use any kind of bones — beef, lamb, chicken, fish.
- Marrow bones make wonderful broth! And don't be afraid to use more terrifying-looking bones like knuckles; these meaty joints are full of gelatine and amino acids, which is exactly what you want.
- You can even use some trimmings and bones from a leftover roast, to get extra use and nutrients from them, while also dramatically reducing your food waste. (It also means you won't need to roast the bones during the first stages of broth-making, as they're already softened and ready to add to your simmering pot.)
- Alternatively, buy raw bones from your butcher; this can be very cost-effective, as you can buy in bulk and freeze some for later.

2 GIVE RAW BONES A GOOD ROASTING

- If using raw bones, a great way to maximise their taste is to brown them first, to lock in their flavours. Melt some extra virgin coconut oil in a large flameproof casserole dish over medium heat. Add the juicy bones and stir to coat them in the oil. Put the lid on and bake for around 30 minutes at 200°C (400°F), until the bones are a gorgeous golden brown. (If you're making chicken broth with a whole chicken, there's no need to brown it first.)

3 ADD VEGIES, AROMATICS & VINEGAR

- Place the pot back on the stove and add some chopped vegies. Onion, parsnip, carrot, celery and garlic are all wonderfully nutritious, and their earthy flavours really enhance the broth.

- You can also add the ends or stalks of vegies, such as the leafy green tops from carrots, to further minimise food waste.
- Stir the vegies, then add plenty of water, preferably filtered, as tap waters can contain heavy metals, which concentrate during boiling.
- Bring to the boil, season with good salt and freshly cracked black pepper, and add any herbs and spices you adore, to make the broth even more flavoursome and supercharged. I love adding bay leaves, healing paprika, and anti-inflammatory turmeric and ginger.
- Also add a good splash of apple cider vinegar, to help draw valuable minerals from the bones.

4 SIMMER AWAY

- Now reduce the heat and leave to simmer, topping up with water as needed. The simmering process draws the gelatine from the bones, making the broth look more like jelly than a liquid stock. In fact, the more jelly-like your broth, the better it is for you — it means you've extracted the maximum amount of goodness!
- Smaller, weaker bones, such as fish bones, only need 1–2 hours of simmering to extract all the mineral goodness, whereas beef, pork and lamb bones will take at least 4–6 hours, or up to a day. The longer you simmer larger, sturdier bones, the more nutrients and gelatine will be released — making your broth wobble even more.
- You can even make the longer-simmering bone broths in a slow cooker, so you don't need to check on them very often.

5 STRAIN, STORE & ENJOY

- When your broth is ready, you can remove any vegies you added (they'll be beautifully soft, ideal for mashing later on), or serve them in the broth, after removing the bones.
- Beef or chicken bones will be easy to remove, but fish broth may contain some soft fine bones, which you'll need to strain out.
- For a clear broth, let it cool, then pass it through a sieve.
- Pour your broth into airtight containers, ready for the fridge or freezer, or freeze in ice-cube trays, for handy portion sizes.
- Please don't discard any fat that solidifies on top — it's a fantastic source of natural healthy fats. It will also help preserve the broth, and is delicious for sautéing vegetables in.
- To use, simply warm the broth and sip on it as a warm drink, or melt a few frozen broth cubes in a pan, to enhance other dishes.

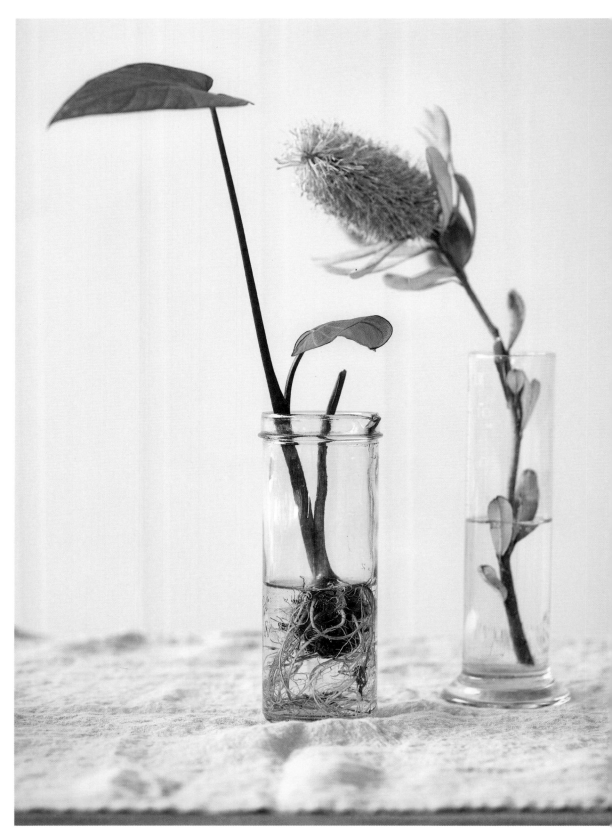

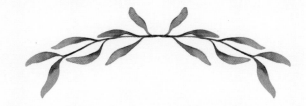

THE SUPERCHARGE YOUR GUT MAINTENANCE PLAN

Now that you understand the inside story of the gut, its connections, and how to support, feed and balance it, it's time to enjoy a host of delicious, healing recipes on the two days each week you are devoting to supercharging your gut.

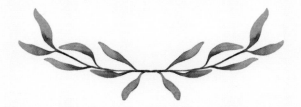

WHY THE MAINTENANCE PLAN WORKS

Before we begin, let's look at how to put all you have learnt about the gut into practice.

LET'S BEGIN WITH THE WHYS

This program works to help reset your gut, and when implemented as a routine two days per week, it's a long-term investment in your health. Why is it so beneficial?

Firstly, you're self-caring. By implementing strategies of stress relief, self-care and rest, you'll be tapping into the gut–brain axis, calming the nervous system and calming your gut. After your two days of self-care, you'll feel lighter and less 'foggy', and see an improvement in your mood and stress levels, which will also improve nerve communication between your brain and gut, optimising digestion and settling digestive troubles such as irritable bowel syndrome.

AND THE WHEREFORES

When you think about the investment you're making, it's a small part of your week for such large benefits. You don't need to follow the program every day; it's more an approach that helps give the terrain and integrity of your gut a boost, so you can live with more vitality and vigour throughout the rest of your week. By giving your body just two days of focused nurturing and nourishment through gut-healing recipes, you'll reset your 'digestive fire', which will allow you to uptake significantly more nutrients from the foods you consume. Your body will be propelled in the week ahead to convert energy more efficiently from within your gut, taking a large load off your digestive system.

AND THEN THE HOW-TOS

Gut-health becomes an enjoyable routine. Just as we brush our teeth every day to prevent nasty trips to the dentist, so too should we implement routines that care for our gut, which is such a vital centre of the body for our overall health. With my Supercharge Your Gut two-day program, you can maintain the health of this amazing system through routines that will become a fun part of your self-care regime.

You'll look forward to trying the new recipes, figuring out which ones you love best, enjoying the mindful routine of cooking and preparing food with love, and routinely dedicating two days a week to gut-nurturing habits, ranging from diet to journalling, digestion-soothing yoga poses, oil-pulling and body brushing (see page 116), and moving your body in a way that's liberating and fun, rather than gruelling and oppressive.

Self-love and self-care don't have to seem like a fairy tale. I've taken all the hard work out of these routines for you. They've all been specifically chosen for their gut-friendly outcomes. All you have to do is put them into action and enjoy the process as well as the benefits.

Are you ready to get started?

HOW TO HEAL YOUR GUT, LAYER BY LAYER

Let's take this step by step — or as I like to put it, layer by layer. The Supercharge Your Gut maintenance plan is a wonderful way to reset the health of your gut through simple, enjoyable recipes and routines that will promote gentle healing and help repair and replenish your digestive health.

The main goal is to give your gut a break from hard-to-digest foods, allowing for repair of the gut lining, lowering inflammation and creating the environment for new strains of healthy microflora to flourish, leading to increased immunity and energy, elimination of pain and bloating, and improved mood.

The program has been designed to give your body the much-needed space to repair as often as you see fit, especially after periods of eating processed foods, drinking alcohol, or living an inflammatory lifestyle that is full of stress, poor health choices or lack of rest. This is a great self-care strategy that will improve your wellbeing and vitality, and its principles can be used as often as you feel you need them.

By nurturing your digestive system two days a week, you'll create environmental changes within your gut that shift the balance of unhealthy microflora to a microbiome that has the capacity to act as a generator of energy in your body. How does it do this? The good guys in your gut actually take a load-bearing role in terms of energy production, turning food into energy at higher rates, and also defending the gut from energy-sapping pathogens that can promote illness and slow you down.

Aside from the routines, recipes and self-care practices that are covered in this book, there are three valuable principles to adhere

to throughout this time of digestive reset that will enhance
the repair of your gut, layer by layer.

1 AVOID FOODS THAT INFLAME THE GUT

Foods that cause inflammation to the gut lining, leaky gut, and
inflammatory immune responses in people with a compromised
gut include:

- alcohol
- gluten (found in wheat, oats, barley, rye, triticale, spelt
  and virtually all processed foods)
- dairy
- caffeine

On your maintenance days, stay away from these foods as much as
possible. By avoiding them you'll be giving your body the best chance
to reset, and you may even find that a range of symptoms you think
are 'normal' actually disappear, bringing a newfound feeling of vitality
and improved digestion.

2 AVOID SUGAR

In my *Heal Your Gut* book and four-week program, stevia is the only
sweetening ingredient used, apart from berries.

For the Supercharge Your Gut maintenance plan, when a recipe
calls for stevia, you can use raw honey or rice malt syrup if you prefer
— without going overboard.

3 BE MINDFUL OF FOOD PAIRING

When you're having belly issues, the way you pair your foods can
have a profound impact on your gut. To maximise your gut's ability
to digest food properly, avoid overloading the system with complex
mixtures of foods. Keep things simple, and follow these tips for
sensible food pairing.

Avoid pairing animal proteins with grains, beans or starchy
vegetables. Each of these foods requires special enzymes to break
them down, and mixing them together can cause chaos for your gut.
Eating animal proteins and starches or grains together causes acid
and alkaline to neutralise one another. In this condition digestive
enzymes can't do their jobs as adequately, digestion is compromised,
and your food begins to ferment. This creates a delicious feast for
candida and pathogenic bacteria.

It's best to combine grains and starchy vegetables with non-starchy land and/or sea vegetables. The best grains to eat are gluten-free and include quinoa, buckwheat, amaranth and millet. Starchy vegetables are pumpkin (winter squash), butternut squash, peas, lima beans, artichokes and sweet potatoes. Non-starchy vegetables include leafy greens, broccoli, asparagus, cauliflower, carrots, bok choy (pak choy), cabbage, celery, lettuce, green beans, garlic, fennel, onions, chives, turnips, sprouts, red radish, yellow squash, zucchini (courgette), cucumber and beetroot (beet).

If grains and starchy vegetables are causing you problems, such as gas and the dreaded belly bulge, you may need to look at more gut healing and an elimination protocol, as covered on pages 70–71.

Avoid consuming large amounts of fats and oils with proteins, as this slows down digestion.

Following these principles will help you to gradually increase your 'digestive fire'. Avoiding inflammatory foods will help to slow down the build-up of toxins in the system, and proper food combining will allow a consistent pattern of easy digestion that will prevent the build-up of undigested food in the gut lining that causes leaky gut and contributes to adverse autoimmune responses.

THE SUPERCHARGE YOUR GUT MAINTENANCE PLAN

So what do I do next, you might be asking? How do I actually maintain good gut health and when do I start?

Having a healthy gut should be something we embrace as part of an ongoing lifestyle plan. There are factors in our everyday modern lifestyles that can sway the balance into favouring an unhealthy gut if we're not willing give our gut a little love and care.

Chemicals and pesticides in our food and water, lack of physical activity due to sedentary jobs, stress, challenged circadian rhythms, overuse of antibiotics — all of these factors have an effect on our microbiome.

The aim of your two Supercharged Gut days each week is to really make a habit of holistic self-care that will reset your biology in a way that supports your microbiome. The information and recipes in this book will guide you through all you need to know, but if you feel you need a bit of extra care and would like to be part of our online community, you can find my Supercharge Your Gut online program at **superchargedfood.com/join-now**

So, let's get started. Choose two days each week to dedicate to supercharging your gut. You can adjust them to suit your lifestyle.

Next, schedule the first week based around the following day plans, remembering that you can switch things around to make it fit in with you. There's a lovely sense of freedom in swapping things around and letting go — it's liberating, so feel free to create your own day plans, based on the ones below.

DAY 1: A WORK DAY

MORNING RITUAL: Wake up early with the sun. Drink a large glass of warm filtered water with the juice of half a lemon or 1 tablespoon apple cider vinegar, to kick-start your liver and hydration. Add a good pinch of Celtic sea salt or Himalayan salt if you have any adrenal issues.

Get outdoors and get moving. The morning sunlight will reset your circadian rhythms and stimulate your pituitary gland to release feel-good hormones, setting you up for a happy day. Ideal exercise forms would be a walk or gentle jog, a gentle yoga class, or swimming.

Shower and switch between bursts of hot and cold water to get your lymphatic system pumping.

While you're in the shower, try oil-pulling. Place 1 tablespoon extra virgin coconut oil or sesame oil in your mouth upon rising, before you've eaten or drunk anything. Swish the oil around your mouth for 10–20 minutes, then spit it out. Never swallow the oil, which will be full of bacteria. Brush your teeth and tongue thoroughly afterwards, to remove any excess oil, or invest in a tongue scraper. Including this simple ritual in your day will offer benefits such as whiter teeth, clearer skin, healthier gums, fresher breath, clearer sinuses, an improved lymphatic system, better sleep and increased energy, and for pre-menopausal women better regulated menstrual cycles.

Dry your skin, then dry body brush in upward strokes towards the heart, and in clockwise circles on your abdomen to improve digestion. Moisturise with coconut or avocado oil if you have some.

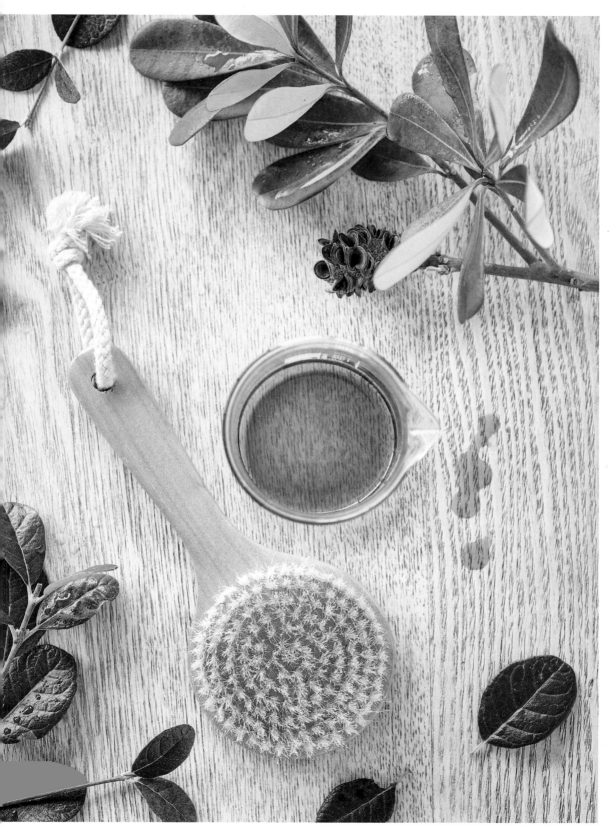

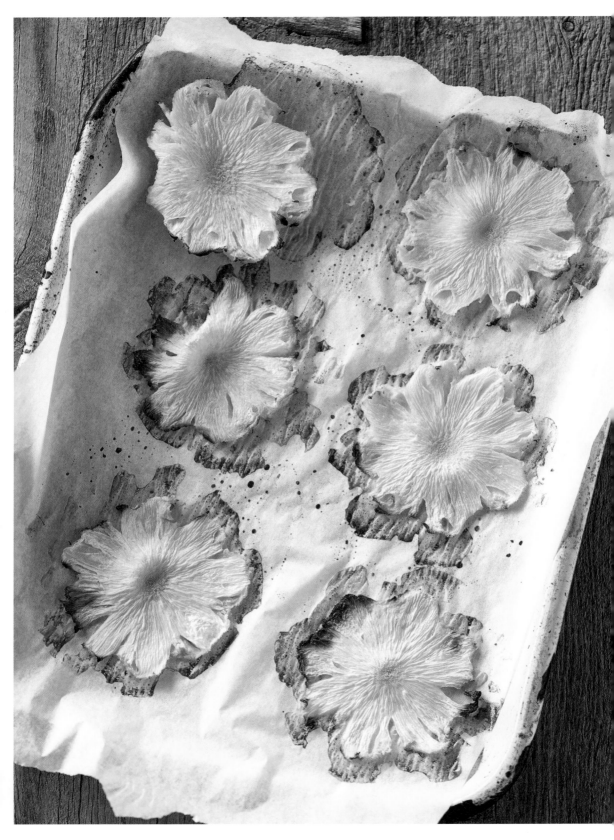

BREAKFAST: Start with some food-grade diatomaceous earth powder (see page 43) in a glass of water. Then try one of the delicious breakfast recipes, or a soothing Maca Maca Maraca (page 150) or Mango & Kale Smoothie Bowl (page 158). If you've prepared a brekkie jar the night before, enjoy that.

THROUGHOUT YOUR DAY: Hydrate! Sip on ginger, lemongrass, fennel and fresh mint teas, pre-make the Hello Vera Smoothie (page 150) and flask it, or enjoy a cup of bone broth (pages 191–198) to soothe the gut lining and aid detoxification. You can also stash pre-made tea mixes in your desk drawer at work, to enjoy throughout the day.

LUNCH: If you simply can't leave your desk at lunchtime, take along an easily digested lunch such as Beef Pho Broth (page 218), Apple & Fennel Soup (page 222), Warm Green Bowl (page 204) or Masala Cauliflower & Peas (page 213). If your gut is ready for fermented food, serve with a side of Cultured Vegetables (page 264).

Pack some 'gut grazers' (page 182–189) if you're prone to snacking — sometimes it's easier to piece together a bunch of snacks than a formal meal. Try the crackers with hommus, tuna dip (or a small tin of tuna), and/or avocado; bring a lemon with you to add a bit of zest.

If you haven't prepared lunch and want to eat out, opt for a soup or stir-fry, or something cooked such as salmon and vegetables.

AT WORK: Instead of sitting and hunching, choose a standing desk if it's available to you. Notice your posture throughout the day and remember to breathe! Go for a walk during your break, or do some yoga poses or stretches to avoid being sedentary, reduce stress and increase focus and productivity. If you really can't leave your desk at lunchtime, please take other short breaks throughout the day.

DINNER: Choose a meal with protein, such as my Thai Fish Curry (page 210) or Seafood Chowder (page 224). Vegetarians can enjoy the Creamy Macadamia, Garlic & Parsnip Soup (page 226) or the easy roasted vegetables in the Prebiotic Tray Bake (page 207).

Make sure you've had enough to eat by indulging in a gut-soothing dessert. Try some Turmeric Fudge (page 279), some Pan-Fried Pineapple with coconut yoghurt (page 282) and, if you're still hungry, finish the night with a Lemon Turmeric Latte (page 141).

EVENING: Introduce an evening ritual to bust stress and soothe digestion. Remember, supporting your gut is all about relaxing the gut and reducing stress. Enjoy a candlelit warm bath with Epsom salts and a soothing essential oil such as lavender to de-stress and relax muscles.

AFTER YOUR BATH: Massage the body with warm oil to improve circulation, activate the lymphatic system and aid detoxification.

Avoid bright lights from screens after the sun goes down, favouring dimmed light, candle light or Himalayan salt lamps.

To wind down on your two gut-healing days every week:

- Read a good book instead of watching TV.
- Journal ten things you were grateful for today.
- Go to bed early!

DAY 2: A WEEKEND OR DAY OFF

6 AM: Wake up naturally with the sun. Drink 500 ml (17 fl oz/2 cups) warm filtered water with lemon juice and a pinch of sea salt.

6.15 AM: Write in a gratitude journal ten things you're thankful for in your life.

6.30 AM: Mix some pure food-grade diatomaceous earth (see page 43), such as my Love Your Gut Powder, in a glass of water and drink it. Then take your yoga mat outdoors if space is available to you (so your eyes and pineal gland have stimulation from the sun) and do at least 30 minutes of yoga or stretching. If you're in the garden or inside, you can use an online video to guide you.

End your practice with a meditation, either guided or self-led, from five minutes to as long as you like.

7.30 AM: Try an Apple Cider Shot (page 147), then make breakfast. It's time to make eggs! Try the Greened-Up Shakshuka (page 165) or Turmeric Scrambled Eggs (page 168), or something different like the Banana Flour Pancakes (page 177).

8 AM: Dry body brushing and oil-pulling (see page 116).

8.30 AM: Shower, using alternate bursts of hot and cold water to increase lymphatic drainage and circulation through the digestive system.

MORNING TEA: Have a slurpie and enjoy it! Don't forget to hydrate during the day with water too.

12 PM LUNCH: Try a pre-digestive. Drink an Olive Oil & Lemon Shot (page 146) to exercise the liver and gallbladder for healthy bile flow before lunch. Then enjoy the Cassava Curry (page 233) or Thai Prawn, Peanut & Zoodle Soup (page 227).

AFTERNOON: Meet up with friends, see a movie, or do an activity you love. Maybe you might like to get into the kitchen and make some of the cleansing treats, such as the Savoury Cupcakes with Pumpkin Mash (page 188) or Apple Cider Gummy Bears (page 276).

AFTERNOON TEA: Enjoy some of your healthy makes and bakes and wash them down with a Virgin Mojito (page 152).

6 PM DINNER: Choose a stew or digestible main. The Prebiotic Tray Bake (page 207) is a lovely choice.

7.30 PM: The three digestive yoga poses outlined on page 95 are optional, but will help restore and calm the gut.

- UTTANASANA (standing forward bend): Calms the nervous system, pacifies the adrenal glands on the kidneys, and compresses the abdominal area to aid digestion.
- PARIPURNA NAVASANA (boat pose): Lifts the diaphragm to take pressure off the stomach and liver, creating space for air to flow through the belly. Pressure on the abdomen aids digestion.
- VIPARITA KARANI (legs up the wall): This restorative pose aids digestion by moving the body into digestive mode.

8.30 PM: Soak in an Epsom salt bath. Afterwards, moisturise and give your belly a gentle massage in a clockwise direction.

9 PM: It's time for your beauty sleep!

YOUR PERSONAL ACTION PLAN

Are you ready to get started? I've got your action plan right here — all you need to do is tweak it and personalise it to suit your own needs.

Whatever inspired you to begin this journey, whether it's an illness, a desire to grow or an eagerness for change in your life, you started this mission for a specific reason. Just as in life, as you travel through this book, not everything I suggest will apply to you and that's okay. Make this book your own. Highlight what you like, use sticky notes for things you want to refer to later, and do whatever you want for it to make total sense to you.

Every single recipe in this book is included for a purpose. I want you to love cooking for your gut. Get inspired and make these recipes your own. Take on a new recipe every week — whether it's a simple tea, or a home-cooked meal.

To get cooking, sometimes you need to think about the way your kitchen runs. Who's the boss of the kitchen in your house? Think about what tools you need to create your favourite recipes and how well you can store the finished dishes. As you know, I love to use mason jars for convenient storage as they don't take up a lot of space. Arrange your kitchen to your advantage and make it your place of support and encouragement.

Create a shopping list and set aside time to go out and shop. To make shopping a little easier, plan your meals for the week on a day that's convenient for you and write down all the ingredients you need. This will save you time and money in the shops and ensure none of the food you buy goes to waste.

I know that changing the contents of your cupboard and fridge can be a lengthy, and sometimes pricey, process. I suggest finding your nearest food store, market or local food community group and checking out the best deals on the foods you need. People are more willing to help than we sometimes realise. All we need to do is ask.

Before we get started, remember that this should never be an unpleasant process. Taking care of your gut is something that should make you feel joyful, not miserable. Clear your calendar, destroy negative thoughts and prepare to nurture and nourish your gut.

Don't be afraid of cooking. One of my favourite things to hear after people read my books is that I've helped them get rid of their fear of the kitchen and allowed them to finally enjoy cooking! Get in the kitchen and enjoy the recipes that you create. Cooking can be a beautiful and therapeutic process if you let it.

If you're having an unyielding craving for a choc-chip muffin coated in frosting, listen to what it may be. What we crave says more about our nutrient requirements than we think. If you're constantly dreaming about sweet foods, you may not be filling your body up with the right nutrients, such as healthy fats or necessary vitamins or minerals. You may also be eating to avoid dealing with emotional issues. Listen to your food clues, think them through and adapt accordingly.

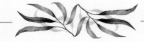

YOUR ACTION PLAN IN A NUTSHELL

- Tailor the plan to your own health goals.
- Get inspired with your favourite recipes.
- Access your kitchen and storage solutions.
- Create a shopping list and set aside time.
- Find your nearest store, market or local food community group.
- Clear your calendar and prepare to nurture and nourish your gut.
- Get into the kitchen and enjoy the recipes.
- Listen to food clues and adapt accordingly.
- Repeat once more each week.

Now you're ready to get underway!

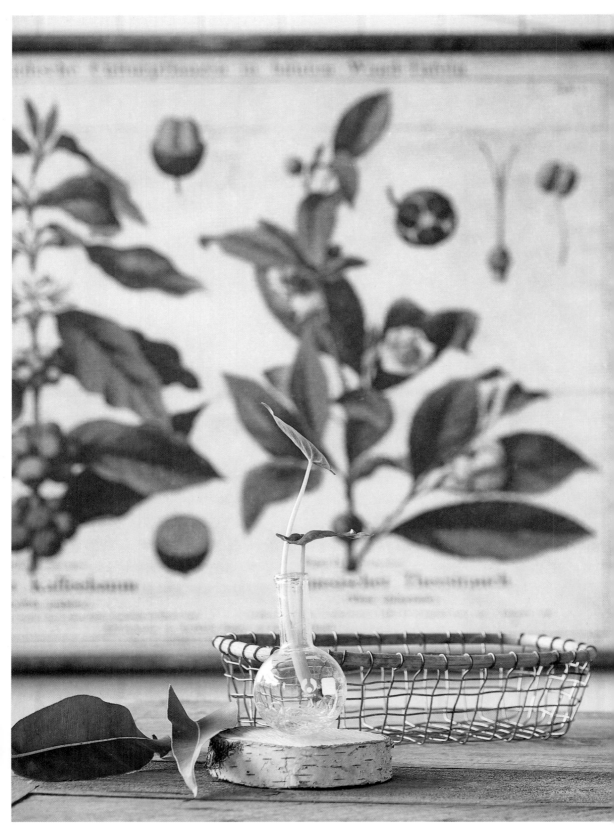

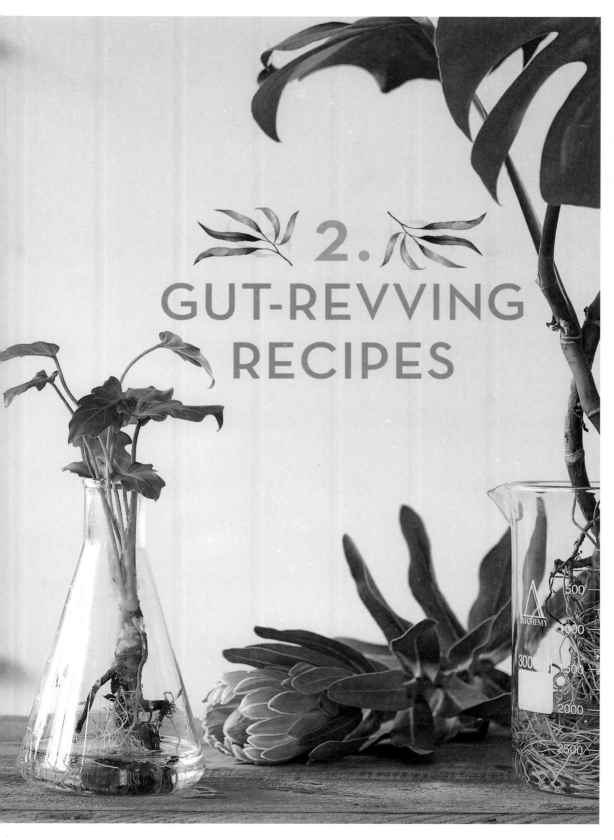

2.
GUT-REVVING
RECIPES

A GUIDE TO THE ICONS

To give your gut the real support it needs, and to help you create a personalised, balanced and nourishing diet, I've included little icons before each recipe so you can ensure it meets your dietary needs. See you later, bloating and tummy trouble!

In some cases you'll need to choose the option for a particular ingredient to suit your individual diet — for example, to make a vegetarian soup, use a vegetable stock rather than a meat broth.

Eating a wide variety of real foods and not cutting out whole food groups unless absolutely necessary is a philosophy that works well for many people in the long term.

Here's a breakdown of what each at-a-glance icon signifies.

● GF GLUTEN-FREE

Gluten is a mixture of proteins found in grains such as wheat, rye, barley and oats. Some people can tolerate oats, but the tricky bit is finding oats that haven't been contaminated by wheat or other grains during processing. Symptoms of gluten sensitivity can include gastrointestinal issues, skin problems, changes in weight, headaches and depression. Gluten sensitivity can make you feel ill or uncomfortable in your gut, and can affect your mood and quality of life.

● WF WHEAT-FREE

Some people find wheat hard for their sensitive gut to digest, and that it can cause allergic reactions. Common symptoms of a wheat allergy can include eczema, hives, asthma, hay fever, irritable bowel syndrome, tummy aches, bloated stomach, nausea, headaches, joint pain, depression, mood swings and tiredness. Wheat products can be replaced with buckwheat, rice, quinoa, tapioca and wheat-free flours.

DF DAIRY-FREE

To avoid dairy in the supermarket, look at labels for any food that contains cow's or goat's milk, cheese, buttermilk, cream, crème fraîche, milk powder, whey, casein, caseinate and margarines, all of which contain milk products. Substitutes for dairy milk can include nut and seed milks, and coconut milk.

SF SUGAR-FREE

Refined sugar can contribute to nutrient deficiencies, as it provides energy without any nutrients. Researchers have reported that people with deficiencies of nutrients such as magnesium, zinc, fatty acids and B-group vitamins are more likely to show symptoms of anxiety and depression.

VEG VEGAN

These recipes contain no meat, eggs, dairy products or honey. To ensure you're obtaining enough of the nutrients needed for optimum health and gut healing, it's a good idea to include forms of protein, and foods containing iron, B12, vitamin D and calcium, in your diet. Good fats from non-meat sources are also very important. Some recipes not marked VEG may still be suitable for lacto-ovo vegetarians — check the ingredient lists.

SHOPPING LIST

Food diversity is vital for a happy and multicultural microbiome. To save you a truckload of time shopping for food, this master shopping list has everything suitable for a gut-friendly pantry. When navigating grocery stores, remember to check labels and bear in mind that everyone is different when it comes to trigger foods, so build up your pantry slowly and see what works for you.

VEGETABLES

Asian greens
Asparagus
Avocados
Bean sprouts
Beetroot (beets)
Bok choy (pak choy)
Broccoli
Brussels sprouts
Butternut pumpkin (squash)
Cabbage
Capsicums (peppers)
Carrots
Cassava
Cauliflower
Celeriac
Celery
Cherry tomatoes
Chillies
Cucumbers
Edamame beans
Eggplants (aubergines)
English spinach
Fennel
Garlic
Green beans
Jerusalem artichokes
Jicama (Mexican yam bean)
Kale
Lettuce
Mushrooms
Olives
Onions
Parsnips
Peas
Plantains
Pumpkin (winter squash)
Rocket (arugula)
Shallots (French and Red Asian)
Silverbeet (Swiss chard)
Snow peas (mangetout)
Spring onions (scallions)
Sprouts (all types)
Squash
Sweet potatoes
Tomatoes
Turnips
Watercress
Zucchini (courgettes)

FRUIT

Apples
Avocados
Bananas
Berries (fresh + frozen)
Lemons
Limes
Mangoes
Papaya
Pineapple

EGGS & MEAT

Beef and veal
Bones for broths
Chicken
Eggs (organic, free-range)
Gelatine
Lamb
Pork

SEAFOOD

Anchovies
Fish (fresh)
Prawns (shrimp)
Salmon (wild-caught)
Sardines
Shellfish
Tuna

MILKS & DRINKS

Coconut cream
Coconut milk
Coconut water (from young coconuts)
Coconut yoghurt
Coffee (decaffeinated)
Dandelion tea
Herbal teas/tisanes
Matcha powder
Nut milks
Teas (decaffeinated)

FATS & OILS

Butter (organic, unsalted)
Cacao butter
Coconut butter
Coconut oil (extra virgin)
Ghee
Olive oil (extra virgin, cold-pressed)
Seed + nut oils (macadamia, walnut, sesame, flaxseed)

SEEDS, NUTS & NUT BUTTERS

Almond butter
Almonds (slivered)
Brazil nut butter
Chia seeds
Flaxseeds (linseed)
Hazelnut butter
Macadamia butter
Nuts (activated)
Pine nuts
Poppy seeds
Pumpkin seeds (pepitas)
Sesame seeds
Sunflower seeds
Tahini

GRAINS, FLOURS & BAKING

Almond meal
Amaranth
Baking powder (gluten- and additive-free)
Banana (plantain) flour
Bicarbonate of soda (baking soda)
Buckwheat
Buckwheat flour
Cacao nibs
Cacao powder (raw)
Coconut (desiccated + flakes)
Coconut flour
Quinoa
Quinoa flakes
Rolled (porridge) oats (gluten-free)
Self-raising flour (gluten-free)
Tapioca flour
Vanilla beans
Vanilla extract (alcohol-free)
Vanilla bean paste
Vanilla powder

HERBS & SPICES

Aleppo pepper
Allspice
Asafoetida
Basil
Black pepper
Cardamom
Chilli (powder + flakes)
Chives
Cinnamon
Cloves
Coriander (cilantro)
Cumin (ground + seeds)
Curry leaves
Curry powder
Dill
Fennel seeds
Fenugreek (leaves + seeds)
Garam masala
Ginger
Kaffir lime leaves
Lemongrass
Marjoram
Mint
Mustard seeds (black + yellow)
Nutmeg
Oregano
Paprika (smoked + sweet)
Parsley
Peppermint oil
Rosemary
Saffron
Sage
Star anise
Sumac
Tarragon
Thyme
Turmeric

CONDIMENTS & SWEETENERS

Apple cider vinegar
Capers
Celtic sea salt
Coconut aminos
Coconut nectar
Coconut sugar
Curry paste
Dijon mustard
Dulse flakes
Fish sauce (gluten-free)
Himalayan salt
Honey (raw)
Kombu
Maca powder
Mustard powder
Nori flakes
Nutritional yeast flakes
Rice malt syrup
Stevia (liquid or powder)
Tamari (wheat-free)
Tamarind (concentrate + purée)
Tomato paste (concentrated purée)
Vegetable stock (sugar- and additive-free)
Yeast flakes (nutritional)

SUPPLEMENTS (OPTIONAL)

Antifungals (caprylic acid, oil of oregano)
Cod liver oil
Collagen (powdered)
Colostrum
Golden Gut Blend (see Note, page 281)
Krill oil
L-glutamine
Licorice root
Love Your Gut Powder (diatomaceous earth)
Magnesium
Probiotics
Slippery elm powder
Zinc

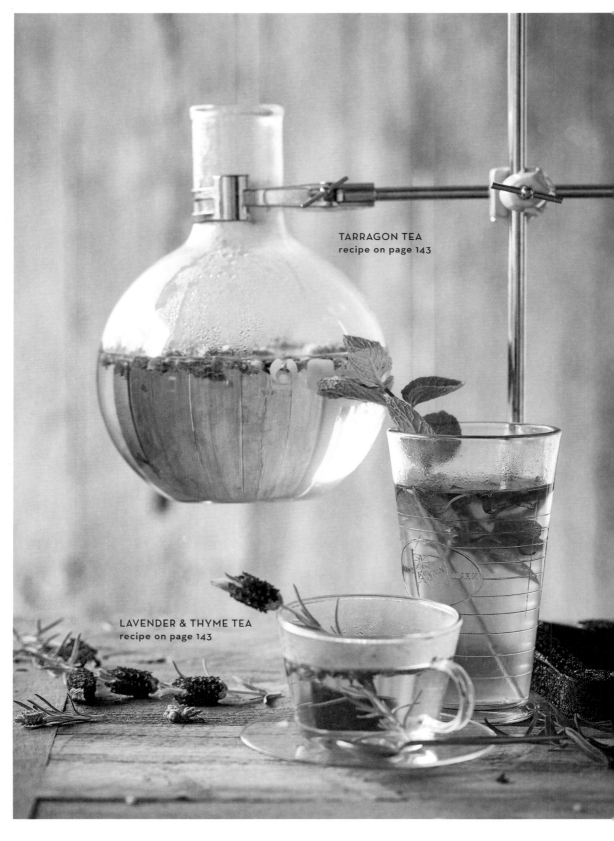

TARRAGON TEA
recipe on page 143

LAVENDER & THYME TEA
recipe on page 143

DRINKS

Introducing smoothies and juices into your day will play a significant role in setting up firm foundations for lifelong health. These potent beverages will infuse vital nutrients, minerals and antioxidants into your gut at top speed, in an easy-to-digest and tasty way. Hello, fibre!

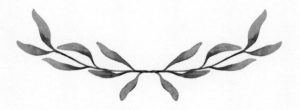

BRAZIL NUT MILK

● GF ● WF ○ DF ● SF ● VEG

MAKES 1 LITRE (35 FL OZ/4 CUPS)

With a creamy dose of good fats, selenium and skin-loving vitamin E, Brazil nut milk makes a great alternative to dairy.

300 g (10½ oz/2 cups) raw Brazil nuts, soaked in filtered water for 3–4 hours, then strained
1 litre (35 fl oz/4 cups) filtered water

6 drops of liquid stevia (optional)
1 teaspoon alcohol-free vanilla extract or vanilla powder

Place all the ingredients in a high-speed blender and whiz until creamy. Pour into a nut milk bag or sieve and strain into a sterilised airtight jug or glass jar. If using a nut milk bag, squeeze the bag until all of the milk is released.

The milk will keep in the fridge for up to 4 days.

MACADAMIA MILK

● GF ● WF ○ DF ● SF ● VEG

MAKES 1 LITRE (35 FL OZ/4 CUPS)

Protein-rich macadamia nuts are a rich source of essential vitamins and minerals, including vitamin A, iron and B vitamins. A gut-loving ingredient, they contain around 7 per cent dietary fibre, both soluble and insoluble. They help you feel satiated and also provide roughage to aid digestion.

155 g (5½ oz/1 cup) raw macadamia nuts, soaked in filtered water for 3–4 hours, then strained
1 litre (35 fl oz/4 cups) warm filtered water

8 drops of liquid stevia, or to taste
¼ teaspoon alcohol-free vanilla extract or vanilla powder

Place all the ingredients in a high-speed blender and whiz for 30 seconds, or until smooth. Pour the milk straight into a sterilised airtight jug or glass jar — it doesn't need to be strained. It will keep in the fridge for up to 4 days.

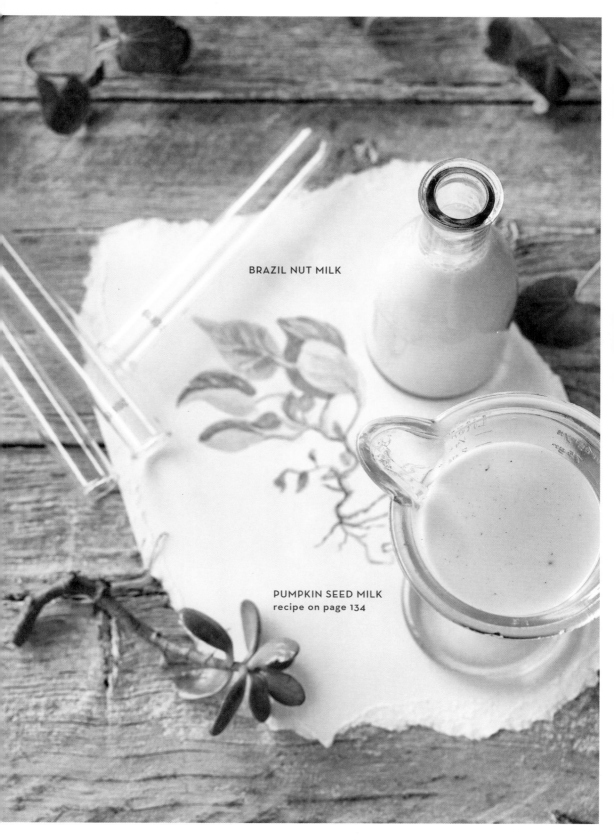

BRAZIL NUT MILK

PUMPKIN SEED MILK
recipe on page 134

PUMPKIN SEED MILK

● GF ● WF ○ DF ● SF ● VEG

MAKES 1 LITRE (35 FL OZ/4 CUPS)

Pumpkin seeds have traditionally been used as an anthelmintic (a substance that helps expel intestinal parasites), and in this gut-healing milk they're teamed up with sesame seeds (from which tahini is made), which have been found to boost the absorption of vitamin E within the gut — helping to prevent inflammation, oxidative stress and chronic disease development.

Sunflower seeds also make a beautifully tasting creamy milk. They're wonderful for aiding DNA repair, and detoxing the body of harmful or damaged cells.

155 g (5½ oz/1 cup) pumpkin seeds (pepitas), soaked in filtered water for 4 hours, then drained
1 teaspoon flaxseed (linseed) meal
1 litre (35 fl oz/4 cups) filtered water

6 drops of liquid stevia
2 tablespoons tahini
1 teaspoon alcohol-free vanilla extract
pinch of Celtic sea salt

Place all the ingredients in a high-speed blender and whiz until creamy.

Pour into a nut milk bag or sieve and strain into a sterilised airtight jug or glass jar. If using a nut milk bag, squeeze the bag until all of the milk is released.

The milk will keep in the fridge for up to 4 days.

 NOTE: *You can use the seed pulp in raw cakes and biscuits, or as a filler in baking. To make **Sunflower Seed Milk**, use soaked sunflower seeds in the recipe above. For extra flavour, you can toast the sunflower seeds before soaking them.*

*You can also try **hemp seed milk** – an excellent choice if you're after a creamy and protein-rich milk that tastes like a blend between cashew and soy. To make this, blend 120 g (4¼ oz/1 cup) of raw hemp seeds with 750 ml (26 fl oz/3 cups) of water and 1 teaspoon of vanilla.*

FLAX MILK

● GF ● WF ○ DF ● SF ● VEG

MAKES ABOUT 1 LITRE (35 FL OZ/4 CUPS)

Flaxseeds may be tiny, but they offer colossal gut-healing benefits. These babies are high in alpha-linolenic acid, an omega-3 fatty acid that can help protect the lining of the digestive tract and is beneficial for people who have Crohn's disease or other significant gut issues.

Replacing your regular nut milk with this variation is a great way to enjoy flax's anti-inflammatory and digestive healing benefits.

3 tablespoons whole flaxseeds (linseeds)
1 litre (35 fl oz/4 cups) filtered water

6 drops of liquid stevia
2 teaspoons alcohol-free vanilla extract

Place all the ingredients in a high-speed blender and whiz until creamy.

Pour into a nut milk bag or sieve and strain into a sterilised airtight jug or glass jar. If using a nut milk bag, squeeze the bag until all of the milk is released.

The milk will keep in the fridge for up to 4 days and is best served chilled. Natural separation may occur; if so, just shake before using.

 NOTE: *Using 'golden' flaxseeds will give a milder flavour.*

CASHEW MILK

● GF ● WF ● DF ● SF ● VEG

MAKES 560 ML (19¼ FL OZ/2¼ CUPS)

Cashew milk is the creamiest, most velvety nut milk on the block. It's mineral rich, providing copper, phosphorus, manganese, magnesium and zinc. Use cashew milk instead of dairy in teas, smoothies, mashes and soups.

165 g (5¾ oz/1 cup) raw cashews, soaked in filtered water for 3–4 hours, then strained
750 ml (26 fl oz/3 cups) filtered water, boiled, then cooled slightly
¼ teaspoon alcohol-free vanilla extract
liquid stevia or stevia powder, to taste

Whiz the cashews, water and vanilla in a high-speed blender until smooth. Strain through a fine sieve, reserving the cashew pulp to use again (see below).

Sweeten the cashew milk with stevia to taste, then pour into a sterilised airtight jug or glass jar.

The milk will keep in the fridge for up to 4 days.

NOTE: *You can make more cashew milk by adding the cashew pulp to the blender with more filtered water; this can be done up to three times. The cashew pulp will keep in a sealed container in the fridge for up to 3 days.*

COCONUT MILK

● GF ● WF ● DF ● SF ● VEG

MAKES 1 LITRE (35 FL OZ/4 CUPS)

It's so easy to make your own coconut milk at home, and you can play around with flavours. For a chocolate or raspberry version, add 2 teaspoons raw cacao powder or a handful of fresh or frozen raspberries when blending.

1 litre (35 fl oz/4 cups) filtered water, boiled, then cooled slightly
130 g (4¾ oz/2 cups) shredded coconut
¼ teaspoon alcohol-free vanilla extract

Place all the ingredients in a high-speed blender and whiz until creamy.

Pour into a nut milk bag or sieve and strain into a sterilised airtight jug or glass jar. If using a nut milk bag, squeeze the bag until all of the milk is released.

The milk will keep in the fridge for up to 3 days. Natural separation may occur; if so, just shake before using.

MASALA CHAI

● GF ● WF ○ DF ● SF ● VEG

MAKES 750 ML (26 FL OZ/3 CUPS)

There's ordinary tea, and then there's chai. Robust and stimulating, masala chai is enjoyed by millions in its native India, and many more all over the world. It's the perfect belly warmer for enhancing and calming the digestive system. All the spices featuring in it have wonderfully unique digestive qualities, in particular cinnamon, which is known for its antifungal and antibacterial properties, making it effective in fighting yeast infections.

4 whole cloves
4 cardamom pods
500 ml (17 fl oz/2 cups) non-dairy milk of your choice,
    such as Coconut Milk (page 137) or Cashew Milk (page 136)
250 ml (9 fl oz/1 cup) filtered water
1 cinnamon stick
½ teaspoon ground ginger, or grated fresh ginger
pinch of freshly cracked black pepper
6 drops of liquid stevia
2 decaffeinated tea bags or dandelion tea bags

Using a mortar and pestle, crush the cloves and cardamom pods slightly, to release their flavours.

Pour the milk and water into a small saucepan. Stir in the crushed spices, cinnamon, ginger, pepper and stevia. Bring to the boil, then remove the pan from the heat.

Add the tea bags, cover the pan and leave to steep for 5 minutes.

Stir, then strain into tea cups and serve.

 NOTE: *If you're suffering from cramps, add ¼ teaspoon fennel seeds to the tea — they're a great anti-spasmodic for the tummy.*

MACA & TAHINI LATTE

● GF ● WF ○ DF ● SF ● VEG

SERVES 1

Unfamiliar with maca? It's the root of a plant that grows in the Peruvian Andes. Packed with vitamins, minerals, essential amino acids and phytochemicals, it tastes like butterscotch and has a nutty, earthy sweetness.

Maca is an adaptogen that supports the adrenal glands, helps regulate hormones and improves energy levels. This nutrient-rich root can be ground into flour and used in baking, or added to smoothies and drinks; you'll find it in supermarkets and health food stores.

This creamy maca latte concoction is a wonderful winter warmer. It makes an excellent coffee substitute in the mornings, and will help to level out your hormones and boost your energy — and even your libido!

250 ml (9 fl oz/1 cup) Coconut Milk (page 137)
2 teaspoons maca powder
1 teaspoon tahini
1 teaspoon alcohol-free vanilla extract or vanilla powder
1 teaspoon rice malt syrup or raw honey, to taste (optional)
toasted sesame seeds, to garnish
ground cinnamon, for sprinkling

Pour the milk into a small saucepan. Add the maca, tahini, vanilla and rice malt syrup, if using. Place over medium heat, whisking until combined and just warm.

Carefully pour into a high-speed blender and whiz for a few seconds until frothy.

Pour into a cup, garnish with sesame seeds and a sprinkling of cinnamon and enjoy.

WARMING GINGER, CARDAMOM & LIME TEA

ZUCCHINI SPICED CUP OF JOY
recipe on page 142

WARMING GINGER, CARDAMOM & LIME TEA

● GF ● WF ○ DF ◐ SF ● VEG

SERVES 1

This zingy tea might catch you off guard when you first try it; if so, add extra sweetener to balance out the flavours. Top with extra lime zest if you like.

375 ml (13 fl oz/1½ cups) filtered water
1 teaspoon grated fresh ginger, or ¼ teaspoon ground ginger
1 tablespoon lemon juice

1 teaspoon lime zest
1 tablespoon lime juice
2 whole cardamom pods, crushed, or ½ teaspoon ground cardamom
6 drops of liquid stevia, or to taste

In a small saucepan, bring the water, ginger, lemon juice, lime zest and lime juice to the boil, stirring well. Remove from the heat, stir in the cardamom, then cover and steep for 3-4 minutes. Strain into a cup and sweeten to taste.

LEMON TURMERIC LATTE

● GF ● WF ○ DF ◐ SF ● VEG

SERVES 1

A lovely latte to help soothe inflammatory gut conditions such as ulcerative colitis. In warmer weather, whiz all the ingredients until frothy, then add ice and serve with a slice of lemon.

250 ml (9 fl oz/1 cup) Coconut Milk (page 137), or other milk of choice
1 teaspoon ground turmeric
¼ teaspoon ground ginger

1 teaspoon vanilla powder
a squeeze of lemon juice
liquid stevia, to taste

Place all the ingredients, except the stevia, in a small saucepan. Bring to the boil, stirring well. Remove from the heat, then cover and steep for 3-4 minutes. Pour into a cup and sweeten to taste.

ZUCCHINI SPICED CUP OF JOY

● GF ● WF ○ DF ● SF

SERVES 1–2

Your gut will be on a joyous high after absorbing the benefits this blend has to offer. Zucchini is often recommended for digestive issues due to its ability to hydrate and top up electrolytes; it also has an anti-inflammatory action within the gastrointestinal tract, reducing flare-ups in leaky gut syndrome, irritable bowel syndrome and ulcer-related symptoms.

The addition of gut-healing, anti-inflammatory spices and gut-wall repairing gelatine makes this recipe a delight for your digestive system.

1 yellow or green zucchini (courgette)
250 ml (9 fl oz/1 cup) Coconut Milk (page 137)
¾ teaspoon ground allspice, plus extra for sprinkling
1 teaspoon ground cinnamon
⅛ teaspoon ground turmeric

a sprinkle of Celtic sea salt
6 drops of liquid stevia
1 teaspoon alcohol-free vanilla extract
1 teaspoon powdered gelatine
whipped coconut cream, to serve (see Note)

Peel the zucchini, then steam until tender. Use a fork to mash the zucchini to a purée consistency, then place in a high-speed blender.

Add the coconut milk, spices, stevia, vanilla and gelatine, and whiz on high until a smooth consistency is reached.

Transfer the mixture to a small saucepan and simmer over low heat for a couple of minutes, stirring and adding more coconut milk if required.

Serve warm, with a dollop of whipped coconut cream and an extra sprinkling of allspice.

 NOTE: *To whip coconut cream, carefully scoop the solid fat from the top of a chilled can of coconut milk or coconut cream (leaving the watery liquid behind), and beat with a hand-held stick blender.*

SUPERCHARGED TIP

Gelatine is a colourless, neutral-tasting thickening agent that forms a jelly when dissolved in water. Gelatine is 35 per cent glycine, an anti-inflammatory amino acid particularly good at healing and soothing the intestinal lining. It's also a great source of arginine, used in many 'fat loss' supplements.

TARRAGON TEA

GF · WF · DF · SF · VEG

SERVES 2

When it comes to gut adoration, tarragon is the paragon of herbs, assisting the digestive process from start to finish — sparking the appetite, increasing salivary flow, and helping the gut produce gastric juices to digest your food. Tarragon also relieves gas, and its powerful antibacterial effects can help in cases of SIBO (small intestinal bacterial overgrowth).

1 tablespoon fresh tarragon leaves
1 teaspoon grated fresh ginger
1 handful of mint leaves
500 ml (17 fl oz/2 cups) boiling
    filtered water

6 drops of liquid stevia, or
    1 teaspoon raw honey (optional)

Put the tarragon, ginger and mint in a teapot and pour in the boiling water. Cover and steep for 5 minutes. Strain into tea cups and sweeten to taste.

LAVENDER & THYME TEA

GF · WF · DF · SF · VEG

SERVES 2

Supercharge your gut with the essential oils of lavender and thyme. These brewable beauties can help alleviate the symptoms of gut dysbiosis, and collaborate with the beneficial bacteria in your tummy.

2 teaspoons unsprayed fresh
    lavender buds, or 1 teaspoon dried
2 teaspoons dried thyme, or
    1 handful of fresh thyme

500 ml (17 fl oz/2 cups) boiling
    filtered water
1 tablespoon lemon juice

Put the lavender and thyme in a teapot. Add the boiling water, then the lemon juice. Cover and allow the herbs to infuse their medicinal oils for 10 minutes.
    Pour into mugs or glasses, or strain the tea if you prefer.

AYURVEDIC CASHEW & CARDAMOM HOT CHOCOLATE

● GF ● WF ● DF ● SF ● VEG

SERVES 2

Try this Ayurvedic twist on the classic hot chocolate, which doubles as a scrumptious indulging ritual as well as a medicinal aid for your gut.

In Ayurvedic tradition, cardamom is considered an excellent digestive that helps minimise gas and bloating. Its soothing, warming effect will help to enhance the absorption of nutrients, as well as calm the nervous system in times of stress.

You could serve this wonderful hot chocolate dusted with extra cinnamon and topped with raw cacao nibs.

500 ml (17 fl oz/2 cups) Cashew Milk (see page 136),
    or milk of your choice
30 g (1 oz/¼ cup) raw cacao powder
1 teaspoon alcohol-free vanilla extract
¼ teaspoon ground cardamom
¼ teaspoon ground cinnamon
pinch of ground nutmeg
pinch of ground ginger
6 drops of liquid stevia, or raw honey to taste

Place all the ingredients in a small saucepan and whisk over low heat until any clumps of cacao and spices have dispersed. Continue stirring as you allow the milk to simmer gently for a few minutes.

Pour into cups and enjoy warm.

 NOTE: *For extra kick, you could add a very small pinch of freshly ground black pepper — as long as spicy foods don't upset your stomach. If you'd like a frothy hot chocolate, whisk or blend just before serving.*

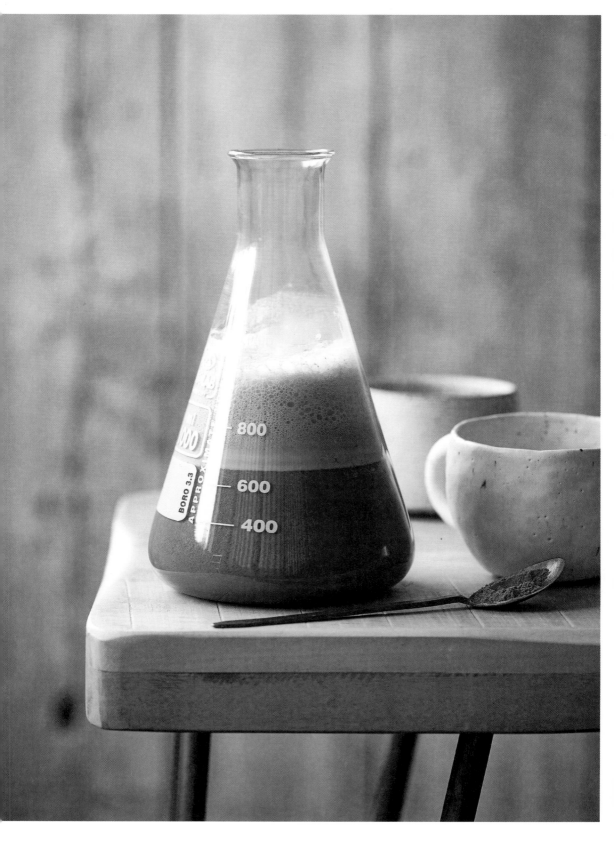

FENUGREEK PRE-DIGESTIVE TEA

● GF ● WF ○ DF ● SF ● VEG

MAKES 500 ML (17 FL OZ/2 CUPS)

Drink this tea before meals as a way to prime the gut for optimum digestion. Fenugreek is well known to aid digestive problems such as upset stomach, gastritis, constipation and inflammatory gut issues.

If you're pregnant, do not consume fenugreek in excess.

500 ml (17 fl oz/2 cups) filtered water
2 teaspoons crushed or ground fenugreek seeds
1/2 teaspoon freshly grated nutmeg
a squeeze of lemon juice
6 drops of liquid stevia, or 1 teaspoon raw honey (optional)

Pour the water into a small saucepan. Add the fenugreek, nutmeg and lemon juice and bring to the boil over medium heat.

Remove from the heat and allow the mixture to steep for 5–7 minutes, or longer if you want a stronger flavour. Strain and sweeten to taste.

OLIVE OIL & LEMON SHOT

● GF ● WF ○ DF ● SF ● VEG

SERVES 1

This glorious shot containing two simple ingredients is the ultimate wake-up call for your gut. Downing this first thing in the morning before breakfast is a great way to flush the gallbladder, kidneys and liver, and promote healthy bile flow. It also helps protect against stomach ulcers and relieve constipation.

juice of 1/2 lemon
2 tablespoons cold-pressed extra virgin olive oil

In a cup, mix together the lemon juice and olive oil. Drink as a detox shot.

APPLE CIDER SHOT

● GF ● WF ○ DF ● SF ● VEG

SERVES 1

Apple cider vinegar has probiotic enzymes to help balance gut bacteria. Try downing this shot around 20 minutes before meals, to improve nutrient assimilation and balance pH levels.

60 ml (2 fl oz/¼ cup) warm filtered water
1 tablespoon apple cider vinegar
1 tablespoon lemon juice
½ teaspoon ground ginger (optional)
6 drops of liquid stevia, or 1 teaspoon raw honey (optional)

Mix all the ingredients together in a small glass and drink before meals to aid digestion. Follow with a little more warm filtered water if needed.

GUT-BALANCING TONIC

● GF ● WF ○ DF ● SF ● VEG

SERVES 2

A soothing tonic to help promote harmony in your inner ecosystem.

1 large carrot
2 celery stalks, trimmed
1 cucumber
½ fennel bulb, chopped
1 lime, peeled
2 cm (¾ inch) knob of fresh ginger, peeled

1 small handful of fresh mint leaves
60 ml (2 fl oz/¼ cup) aloe vera juice
250 ml (9 fl oz/1 cup) coconut water
1 probiotic capsule (optional)
5 drops of liquid stevia, or 1 teaspoon raw honey (optional)
ice cubes, to serve

Roughly chop the carrot, celery, cucumber and fennel, then place in a high-speed blender. Add the lime, ginger and mint leaves and whiz until smooth. Stir in the aloe vera juice, coconut water and the contents of the probiotic capsule, if using. Sweeten to taste and serve immediately, over ice.

PRE-DIGESTIVE GREEN SHOT

APPLE CIDER SHOT
recipe on page 147

OLIVE OIL & LEMON SHOT
recipe on page 146

PRE-DIGESTIVE GREEN SHOT

● GF   ● WF   ○ DF   ● SF   ● VEG

SERVES 2–3

Full of bile-moving ingredients such as parsley and granny smith apples, this green shot is the ultimate cholagogue, or bile mover. Bile production is one of the most critical processes in nutrient absorption and for breaking down fats, and this shot acts like a solvent on stagnant bile in the liver, helping the detoxification process.

250 ml (9 fl oz/1 cup) filtered water
2 tablespoons lemon juice
6 celery stalks, trimmed and
   chopped
45 g (1½ oz/1 cup) baby English
   spinach leaves

4 granny smith apples, cut into
   wedges
5 cm (2 inch) knob of fresh ginger,
   peeled
1 handful of parsley, including
   the stems

Pour the water and lemon juice into a high-speed blender. Add the remaining ingredients and whiz until smooth.

If you prefer a shot with no pulp, just pour the mixture through a fine-mesh sieve and strain it into a jar.

Drink as a pre-digestive shot before meals.

You can keep the pulp and whiz it into soups or pancake mixes.

MACA MACA MARACA

● GF ● WF ○ DF ● SF ● VEG

SERVES 2

This deliciously healing smoothie, worth making part of your essential weekly ritual, unites the balancing properties of maca with light and creamy macadamia milk, encompassing tummy moisturising healthy fats, as well as the minerals selenium, iron, magnesium and zinc. Twinning!

250 ml (9 fl oz/1 cup) Macadamia Milk (see page 132)
1 teaspoon maca powder

½ teaspoon alcohol-free vanilla extract or vanilla bean paste
a few drops of liquid stevia, to taste

Place all the ingredients in a high-speed blender and whiz until smooth. Pour into glasses or jars and serve.

HELLO VERA SMOOTHIE

● GF ● WF ○ DF ● VEG

SERVES 2

Say hello to digestive bliss with this soothing smoothie. You can serve this one over ice cubes, if you like.

250 ml (9 fl oz/1 cup) Almond Milk (see Note, page 153) or Coconut Milk (page 137)
125 ml (4 fl oz/½ cup) pure aloe vera juice
80 g (2¾ oz/½ cup) fresh or frozen organic blueberries

½ large ripe banana, or 1 small lady-finger banana
2 teaspoons extra virgin coconut oil
1 handful of basil leaves, plus extra to garnish
liquid stevia, to taste (optional)

Place all the ingredients in a high-speed blender and whiz until smooth. Pour into glasses or jars, garnish with extra basil and serve.

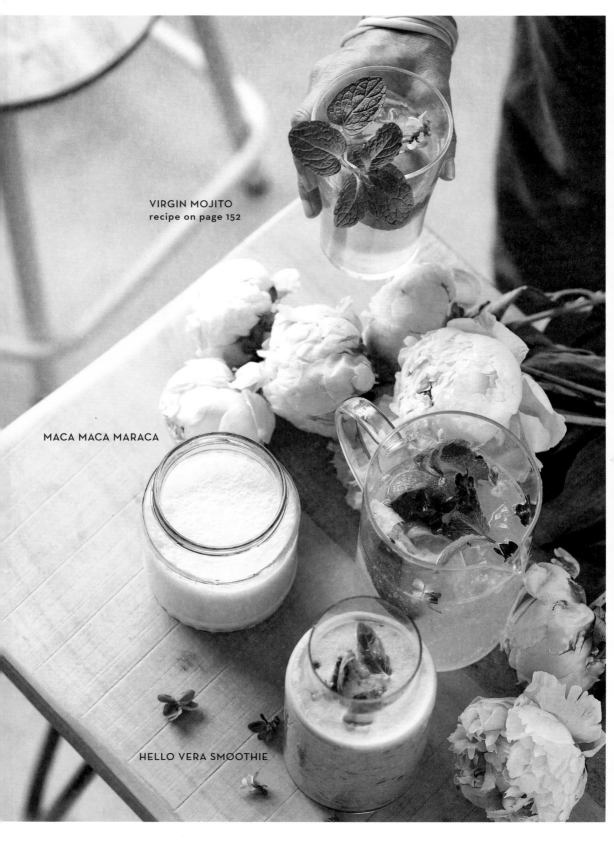

VIRGIN MOJITO
recipe on page 152

MACA MACA MARACA

HELLO VERA SMOOTHIE

VIRGIN MOJITO

● GF ● WF ● DF ● SF ● VEG

SERVES 4

There's no need to cry through 'dry July' with this hangover-free baby up your sleeve. This mojito is the perfect way to be the life of the party, sans alcohol, and will provide an abundant hit of liver-loving ingredients, rather than burdening your most important detox organ.

This mojito makes great popsicles, too — just replace the mineral water with coconut water. See the popsicle recipes on pages 288–289.

2 limes
1 handful of mint leaves, plus extra to garnish
6 drops of liquid stevia
1 litre (35 fl oz/4 cups) mineral water
crushed ice, to serve

Grate the zest from one of the limes and place it in a large jug. Cut the zested lime into thin wedges and add to the jug with the mint and stevia. Cut the other lime into wedges and set aside for serving.

Pour about 250 ml (9 fl oz/1 cup) of the mineral water into the jug. With a long-handled spoon or muddler, mash or stir the mixture gently, then leave to infuse for about 10 minutes.

Pour into tall glasses, then top up each glass with the remaining mineral water. Top with crushed ice and the reserved lime wedges. Garnish with extra mint and serve.

HAPPY-GUT MANGO SMOOTHIE

● GF   ● WF   ○ DF   ● VEG

SERVES 1

This recipe is a beauty if you're looking to increase your intake of
iron in a form that's readily absorbed and doesn't cause constipation.
The diatomaceous earth contains absorbable iron, and the vitamin C
in the mango can help with its absorption.

1 frozen banana
1 small handful of frozen mango chunks
250 ml (9 fl oz/1 cup) Almond milk (see Note), or other
    milk of your choice
1 teaspoon food-grade diatomaceous earth (see page 43),
    such as my Love Your Gut Powder (optional)
½ teaspoon alcohol-free vanilla extract or vanilla powder
pinch of ground cinnamon
pinch of ground nutmeg
½ teaspoon ground turmeric

Place all the ingredients in a high-speed blender and whiz until smooth.
Pour into a tall glass and enjoy.

NOTE: *To make 1 litre (35 fl oz/4 cups) **Almond Milk**, soak 160 g (5¾ oz/
1 cup) raw almonds in filtered water for 3–4 hours, then strain and add to a
high-speed blender with 1 litre (35 fl oz/4 cups) warm filtered water, 8 drops
of liquid stevia (or to taste) and ¼ teaspoon alcohol-free vanilla extract or
vanilla powder. Whiz until smooth. Pour through a strainer, into a sterilised
airtight jug or glass jar. The milk will keep in the fridge for up to 4 days. For
a very pale milk, you can use blanched almonds instead of raw almonds.*

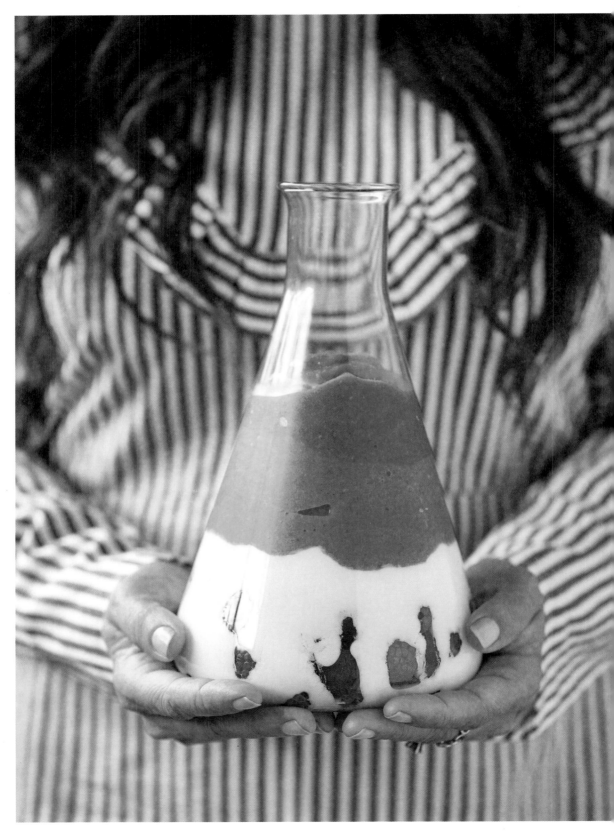

RASPBERRY & COCONUT YOGHURT SLURPIE

● GF ● WF ○ DF ● VEG

SERVES 2

Wave goodbye to memories of convenience-store slurpies and welcome in a blend made with luscious coconut yoghurt and sweet raspberries. This slurpie is full of friendly bacteria to build up your microbial team, paired with immune-boosting antioxidant-rich berries to create an environment in the gut that is resilient against pathogens.

100 g ($3\frac{1}{2}$ oz) frozen raspberries
1 frozen banana, cut into chunks
juice of $\frac{1}{2}$ lemon
fresh raspberries, to serve
250 g (9 oz) coconut yoghurt
1 teaspoon vanilla powder

Place the frozen raspberries, banana and lemon juice in a high-speed blender and whiz until smooth. (If you like, you can spread the mixture on a tray and freeze for 10–30 minutes, or simply serve as is.)

Divide the fresh raspberries and half the yoghurt between two serving glasses. Sprinkle with the vanilla powder. Add the remaining yoghurt, top with the frozen slurpie mixture and serve.

SUPERCHARGED TIP

*For a **Mint Slice** version, replace all the raspberries with a handful of mint leaves, 1 tablespoon cacao nibs, 1 tablespoon tahini and 1 tablespoon chia seeds. For a mouthwatering **Lemon Meringue** version, use 2 tablespoons lemon juice and 1 teaspoon lemon zest instead of the raspberries. See page 107 for more tips on creating slurpie magic in your kitchen.*

MOCHA & BANANA SMOOTHIE BOWL

● GF ● WF ○ DF ● VEG

SERVES 1

People will be wondering what has you so chirpy early in the day! Made with coffee, raw cacao, chia seeds and hazelnuts, with fruity hums of banana, this delectably thick, chocolatey smoothie bowl will give you a natural hit of dopamine — the 'happy' hormone. Think about all the good fats and complex carbohydrates found in banana and nuts, then times them by two, and you'll find yourself powering through your day like a Russian gymnast, performing effortless backflips, half turns and triple twists.

30 ml (1 fl oz) shot of espresso coffee or dandelion tea
1 tablespoon chia seeds
2 tablespoons raw cacao powder
1 tablespoon food-grade diatomaceous earth (see page 43), such as my Love Your Gut Powder (optional)
1 frozen banana, sliced

40 g (1½ oz/¼ cup) hazelnuts (or any nuts of your choice), soaked and roasted
125 ml (4 fl oz/½ cup) Coconut Milk (page 137)
125 ml (4 fl oz/½ cup) Almond Milk (see Note, page 153), or other non-dairy milk of your choice
toppings of your choice, to serve

Pour the coffee or dandelion tea into a small bowl, add the chia seeds and let them sit for a few minutes. Transfer to a high-speed blender.

Add the cacao powder, diatomaceous earth (if using), banana and hazelnuts. Pour in the coconut milk and almond milk and whiz until there are no lumps; the mixture can be quite thick. If your blender is struggling, add extra almond milk or water in small amounts to help it along.

Pour the smoothie into a bowl or serving vessel; we've used half a coconut shell. Garnish with your choice of toppings — fresh banana slices, a sprinkling of mixed nuts and seeds, shaved fresh coconut, micro herbs — and dig in!

SUPERCHARGED TIP

The great thing about a smoothie bowl is that you can add any type of sneaky green, and never taste the difference. Try a handful of baby English spinach, kale, avocado or even frozen peas, to get a headstart on your vegie intake for the day. PS: You don't need to add the coffee if you don't want to — or you can use a decaffeinated version instead.

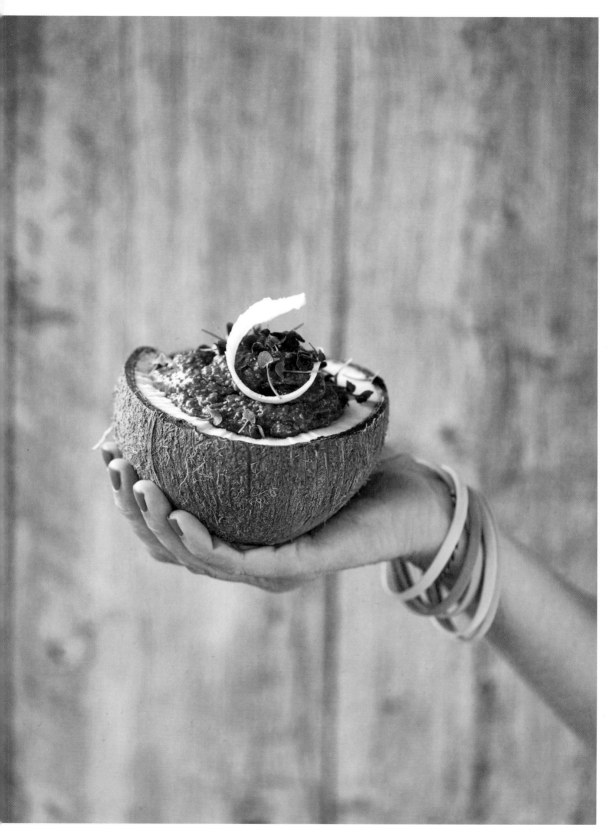

MANGO & KALE SMOOTHIE BOWL

● GF ● WF ○ DF ● VEG

SERVES 2

Smoothie bowls are simply a thicker version of a smoothie — like those thickshakes you may have enjoyed as a child, which you could barely suck through a straw without getting fish face.

Here's a much more nourishing blend to be enjoyed with a spoon, bursting with phytonutrients and enzymes that'll give you an easily digested energy boost for the day ahead.

Serve with your choice of toppings — fresh passionfruit, extra flaxseeds or chia seeds, flaked coconut, fresh berries.

½ ripe avocado
2 frozen bananas, cut into chunks
1 fresh mango, roughly chopped, or 1 large handful
    of frozen mango chunks
2 large handfuls of baby English spinach
2 kale leaves, centre spines and stems removed
375 ml (13 fl oz/1½ cups) Coconut Milk (page 137)
    or Almond Milk (see Note, page 153)
1 tablespoon flaxseed (linseed) meal
1 tablespoon tahini

Place all the ingredients in a high-speed blender and whiz until creamy and smooth. Add more milk to thin the smoothie a little, if necessary.

Scoop into two serving bowls and add your favourite toppings.

SUPERCHARGED TIP

Having a stash of frozen bananas means you'll always have a sustaining smoothie bowl on offer, allowing you to whiz up a deliciously customised blend of fibre-rich vegetables and fruit, bejewelled with different crunchy sprinkles such as cacao nibs, nuts, seeds and/or coconut.

RASPBERRY & CHIA OVERNIGHT BREKKIE JAR

● GF ● WF ○ DF ● VEG

SERVES 1

Cue these ingredients the night before and take the hectic out of morning rush hour.

1 small handful of fresh or frozen raspberries, plus extra to serve
1 small handful of fresh or frozen organic blueberries, plus extra to serve
pinch of vanilla powder
pinch of ground cinnamon

3 tablespoons coconut flakes
3 tablespoons chia seeds
250 ml (9 fl oz/1 cup) non-dairy milk of your choice; Almond Milk (see Note, page 153) is nice
1 tablespoon nut butter (optional)

Combine the berries, vanilla, cinnamon, coconut and chia seeds in a mason jar. Gently mash the berries, then stir in the milk. Pop the lid on and leave in the fridge overnight. Serve topped with the nut butter and extra berries.

MAX (MANGO, SESAME & FLAX) BREKKIE JAR

● GF ● WF ○ DF ● SF ● VEG

SERVES 2

Take it to the max and eat your heart out with this breakfast in a jar! Optional toppings include toasted sesame seeds, fresh mango and flaked coconut.

2 teaspoons flaxseed (linseed) meal
1 fresh mango, chopped, or 1 large handful of frozen mango chunks
2 tablespoons tahini
2 tablespoons coconut yoghurt
1/2 teaspoon ground cinnamon

pinch of ground nutmeg
small pinch of Celtic sea salt (optional)
250 ml (9 fl oz/1 cup) Coconut Milk (page 137), or other milk of your choice

Place all the ingredients in a high-speed blender and whiz until smooth. Pour into two mason jars or serving glasses and enjoy.

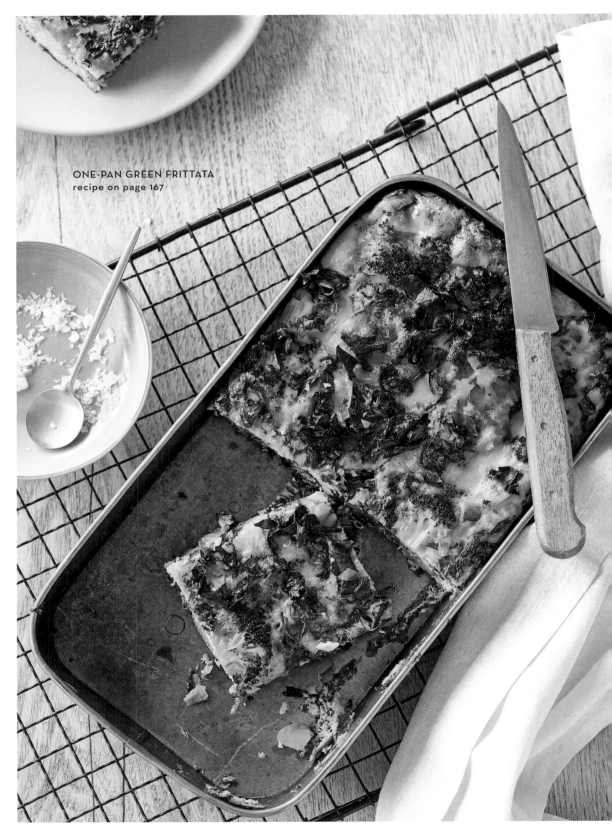

ONE-PAN GREEN FRITTATA
recipe on page 167

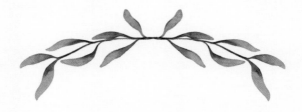

NOURISHING BREAKFASTS

Set your gut up for a supercharged day with shakshuka two ways, glorious gutmeal or creamy chocolate zoats. From sweet to savoury, this chapter has all your breakfast bases covered.

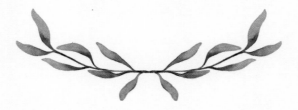

CRUSTLESS VEGETABLE QUICHE

● GF　● WF　● DF　● SF

SERVES 4

Enjoy this gut-friendly twist on the classic French quiche with a side of fresh greens. This *petit plaisir* is a lovely dish to throw together on the weekend, to cut into convenient portions for delicious packed lunches throughout the week. Eggs provide the perfect proportion of fats, proteins, vitamins and minerals needed to sustain you throughout your day.

8 free-range eggs
125 ml (4 fl oz/½ cup) Almond Milk (see Note, page 153)
1 handful of basil leaves
1 thyme sprig, leaves picked
½ teaspoon ground cumin
½ teaspoon Celtic sea salt
2 tablespoons nutritional yeast flakes
10 asparagus spears, cut into 2.5 cm (1 inch) lengths and lightly sautéed
1½ cups sautéed chopped mixed vegetables, such as leek, red onion,
　　garlic, baby English spinach, zucchini (courgette), red capsicum (pepper),
　　cherry tomatoes and rocket (arugula)
mint leaves, to garnish (optional)

Preheat the oven to 180°C (350°F). Grease a 22 cm (8½ inch) pie dish or ovenproof frying pan.

Whisk the eggs well in a large bowl, then whisk in the almond milk, herbs, cumin, salt and yeast flakes.

Evenly scatter the asparagus and sautéed vegetables around the pie dish and pour the egg mixture over the top.

Transfer to the oven and bake for 25–30 minutes, or until the quiche is set in the middle and the top is puffy and lightly browned.

Enjoy warm or at room temperature, garnished with mint if desired.

SUPERCHARGED TIP

This is a great way to use up any vegetables you have sitting in the fridge.

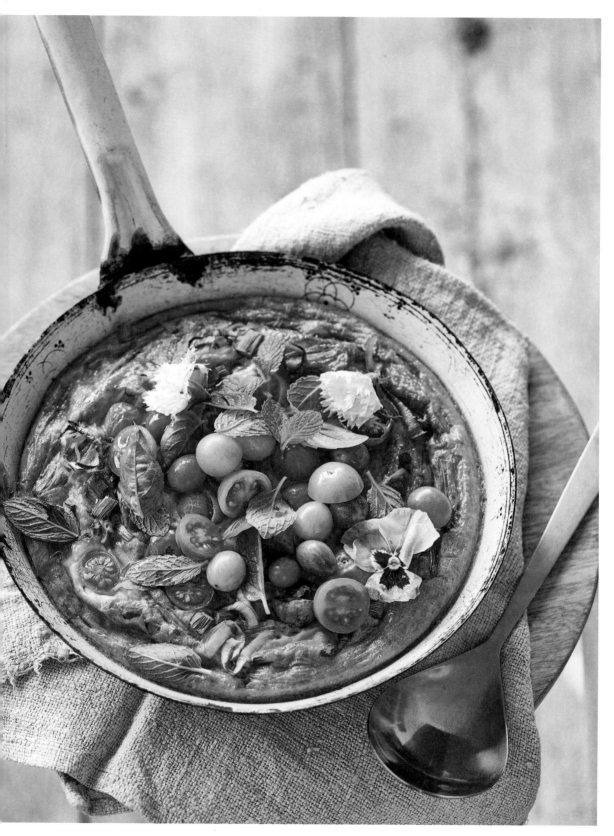

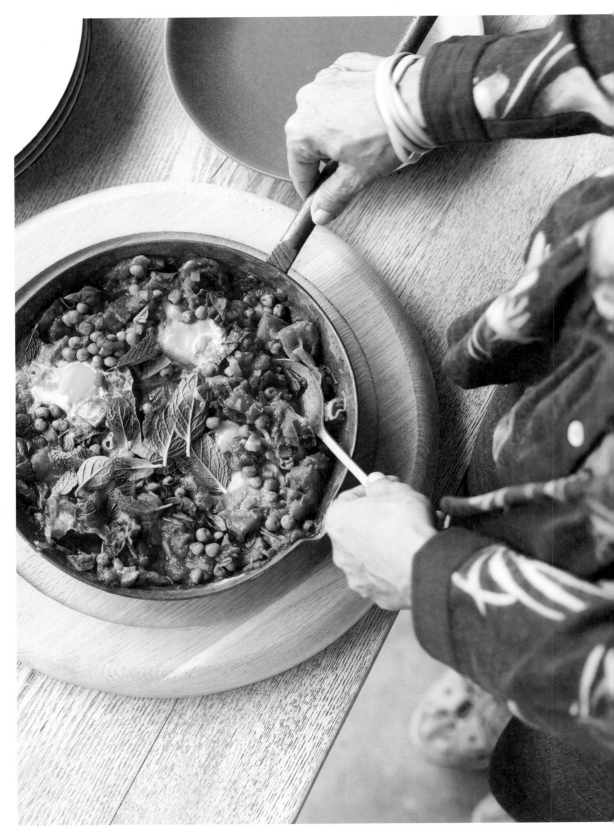

GREENED-UP SHAKSHUKA

● GF ● WF ○ DF ● SF

SERVES 4 GENEROUSLY

Shakshuka celebrates the flavours of the Middle East and North Africa, and is one of my favourite ways to jazz up the humble egg. Loaded with medicinal spices and bursting with lycopene, this tomatoey one-pan wonder won't fail to impress. It's a beautiful way to enjoy a communal breakfast with loved ones.

2 tablespoons olive oil
1 leek, white part only, washed well and sliced
3 garlic cloves, peeled and thinly sliced
1 green capsicum (pepper), diced
pinch of chilli powder or paprika
1 teaspoon ground cumin or cumin seeds
3 fresh bay leaves

1 teaspoon tomato paste (concentrated purée)
800 g (1 lb 12 oz) tinned chopped tomatoes
250 g (9 oz/1¾ cups) frozen peas
1 large handful of baby English spinach leaves
4 large free-range eggs
mint leaves, to garnish

Heat the olive oil in a large frying pan over high heat.

Add the leek, garlic, capsicum, spices and bay leaves and cook, stirring often, for 5 minutes, or until the capsicum is softened and the spices are fragrant.

Stir in the tomato paste, tinned tomatoes and peas, then bring to the boil.

Reduce the heat to low, season to taste with sea salt and freshly ground black pepper and cook for 5 minutes, or until the peas are nearly done. Stir in the spinach.

Make four divots in the sauce and crack an egg into each one. Cover and leave for about 3–5 minutes, or until the eggs are cooked to your liking; the yolks should still be soft.

Serve straight from the frying pan, garnished with mint leaves.

 NOTE: *For a beefed-up shakshuka, use 2 red capsicums rather than 1 green one. After sautéing the vegies, add 300 g (10½ oz) minced (ground) beef and brown it in the pan, breaking up any lumps and letting it cook through. Instead of mint, top the shakshuka with chopped coriander (cilantro).*

GREEN PIKELETS

● GF ● WF ○ DF ● SF

SERVES 2

Is a Sunday morning really a Sunday morning without pikelets?

When I reminisce about some of my favourite Sunday mornings, they always seem to involve late mornings, lazy tunes, light rain, and steaming hot pikelets with toppings galore!

After years of experimenting, I've finally come up with a gut-friendly pikelet recipe I know you'll love.

250 g (9 oz) bunch of English spinach, leaves roughly chopped
3 tablespoons chia seeds
50 g (1¾ oz/½ cup) almond meal
2 free-range eggs
1 tablespoon smooth nut butter
1 tablespoon food-grade diatomaceous earth (see page 43),
   such as my Love Your Gut Powder (optional)
1 teaspoon ground cinnamon
170 ml (5½ fl oz/⅔ cup) Almond Milk (see Note, page 153),
   or other milk of your choice
good pinch of Celtic sea salt
1 tablespoon extra virgin coconut oil

Place all the ingredients, except the coconut oil, in a food processor and blitz until smooth. Let the batter rest for 5–10 minutes.

Heat a frying pan over medium heat and add half the coconut oil.

Using 2–3 tablespoons of batter for each pikelet, cook them in batches for 5 minutes on one side, then flip them over and cook the other side for about 3 minutes.

Transfer the pikelets to a plate and keep warm while cooking the remaining batter.

Serve warm, with your favourite toppings.

ONE-PAN GREEN FRITTATA

● GF ● WF ○ DF ● SF

SERVES 4–6

I really do enjoy a good one-pan dish, and this green frittata scores high on both simplicity and supercharged goodness. I'll take any opportunity to cram more greens into my day, and this frittata is loaded with spring onions, spinach, kale and broccoli — all rich in micronutrients and compounds important for cleansing the gut, and giving a bile-moving blessing to your liver.

1 head of broccoli, chopped into florets
2 tablespoons extra virgin olive oil, plus extra to serve
3 spring onions (scallions), chopped
45 g (1½ oz/1 cup) baby English spinach leaves
3 kale leaves, centre spines and stems removed, then chopped
½ teaspoon ground cumin
1 teaspoon grated lemon zest
1 teaspoon lemon juice
12 free-range eggs, whisked
2 tablespoons nutritional yeast flakes

Preheat the oven to 190°C (375°F).

Bring a saucepan of water to the boil. Add the broccoli and blanch for 3–5 minutes, or until tender–crisp. Drain and set aside.

Heat the olive oil in an ovenproof frying pan over medium heat, then cook the spring onion for a few minutes, until softened.

Add the broccoli, spinach and kale and sauté for about 3 minutes, or until softened. Stir in the cumin, lemon zest and lemon juice.

Pour the eggs over, sprinkle with the nutritional yeast and transfer the pan to the oven. Bake for 30 minutes, or until the eggs are set and golden.

Carefully remove the pan from the oven — the handle will be hot! Dress with an extra drizzle of olive oil and a sprinkling of sea salt and serve.

TURMERIC SCRAMBLED EGGS

Eggs and turmeric are a match made in heaven. Here are two simple ways to enjoy a sprinkling of turmeric's golden medicinal magic.

● GF ● WF ○ DF ● SF

SERVES 2

2 tablespoons extra virgin olive oil
  or coconut oil
3 garlic cloves, crushed
1 small brown onion, chopped
4 free-range eggs, whisked
1 tablespoon wheat-free tamari

½ teaspoon ground cumin
2 teaspoons ground turmeric,
  or to taste
2 tablespoons nutritional yeast
  flakes
basil or mint leaves, to serve

Heat the oil in a frying pan over medium heat. Sauté the garlic and onion for about 5 minutes, or until the onion is translucent.

Add the eggs and stir, then add the tamari, cumin and turmeric. Cook for about 3–4 minutes, stirring continuously.

Sprinkle with the nutritional yeast, tear the herbs over and serve.

TURMERIC PICKLED EGGS

● GF ● WF ○ DF

SERVES 3

250 ml (9 fl oz/1 cup) apple cider
  vinegar
pinch of Celtic sea salt
1 teaspoon coconut sugar

2 teaspoons ground turmeric
6 free-range eggs, hard-boiled,
  cooled and peeled
2 garlic cloves, thinly sliced

In a saucepan, bring the vinegar, salt, sugar, turmeric and 125 ml (4 fl oz/½ cup) filtered water to a gentle simmer.

Place the eggs in a mason jar with the garlic. Pour the vinegar mixture over them and leave to cool. Screw the lid on and refrigerate for 1–3 days.

The pickled eggs are lovely cut in half and sprinkled with sea salt for a snack.

TURMERIC PICKLED EGGS

TURMERIC SCRAMBLED EGGS
served with crackers from page 184

BANANACADO BREAD

● GF ● WF ○ DF

MAKES 1 LOAF

Never let an over-ripe banana go to waste; stash it in the freezer to add a quick creaminess to smoothie bowls and drinks.

This banana and avocado bread is a beautiful way to combine two everyday superstar ingredients straight from the fruit bowl. Skip the café variety that's crammed with wheat and sugar, and share a few slices of this around on a morning coffee break to score instant workplace applause.

Diatomaceous earth is an optional addition, but a worthwhile way to sneak in some gut-healing, detoxification and extra minerals that will add lustre to your skin, hair and nails.

3 large over-ripe bananas, peeled
$1/2$ large avocado, or $3/4$ small avocado
3 free-range eggs
2–4 tablespoons rice malt syrup, to taste
200 g (7 oz/2 cups) almond meal
3 tablespoons food-grade diatomaceous earth (see page 43),
    such as my Love Your Gut Powder (optional)
1 teaspoon baking powder (gluten- and aluminium-free)
$1/4$ teaspoon bicarbonate of soda (baking soda)

Preheat the oven to 160°C (315°F). Line an 11 x 21 cm ($4^{1}/4$ x $8^{1}/4$ inch) loaf (bar) tin with baking paper.

Place the banana and avocado in a high-speed blender and whiz until smooth, or mash together with a fork if you'd like a more rustic, chunky bread.

Add the eggs and rice malt syrup and mix well.

In a separate bowl, combine the remaining ingredients, then stir them through the banana mixture until combined.

Spoon the batter into the loaf tin and bake for 55–60 minutes, or until a skewer inserted into the middle comes out clean.

Leave to cool before turning out of the tin. The loaf will keep in an airtight container in the fridge for up to 3 days, or can be frozen for up to 2 weeks.

APPLE & CINNAMON OAT BOWL

● GF ● WF ○ DF ● VEG

SERVES 2

This is such a lovely calming way to begin the day. When autumn hits, there's something comforting and ritualistic about warming your hands around a bowl of hot creamy porridge. As an added benefit, oats are high in manganese, magnesium and soluble fibre — a fabulous way to keep your digestion calm and regular.

Great toppings include fresh raspberries (or thawed frozen ones), hemp seeds, nut butter, coconut yoghurt and Fermented Berries (see page 268). Instead of oats, you can use quinoa or buckwheat if you prefer.

3 green apples, peeled and sliced
1½ teaspoons ground cinnamon, plus extra for sprinkling
60 ml (2 fl oz/¼ cup) filtered water
95 g (3¼ oz/1 cup) organic gluten-free rolled (porridge) oats
500 ml (17 fl oz/2 cups) Coconut Milk (page 137)
¼ teaspoon vanilla powder

Place the apples, cinnamon and water in a small saucepan and bring to the boil, then reduce the heat and simmer for 7–10 minutes, or until the apples are soft. Remove from the heat.

Meanwhile, in another saucepan, simmer the oats in the coconut milk for 12–15 minutes, or until the oats are tender, stirring regularly.

Stir the apples and vanilla powder through the oats and continue cooking for another 1–2 minutes.

Spoon into serving bowls, sprinkle with extra cinnamon and add any toppings of your choice.

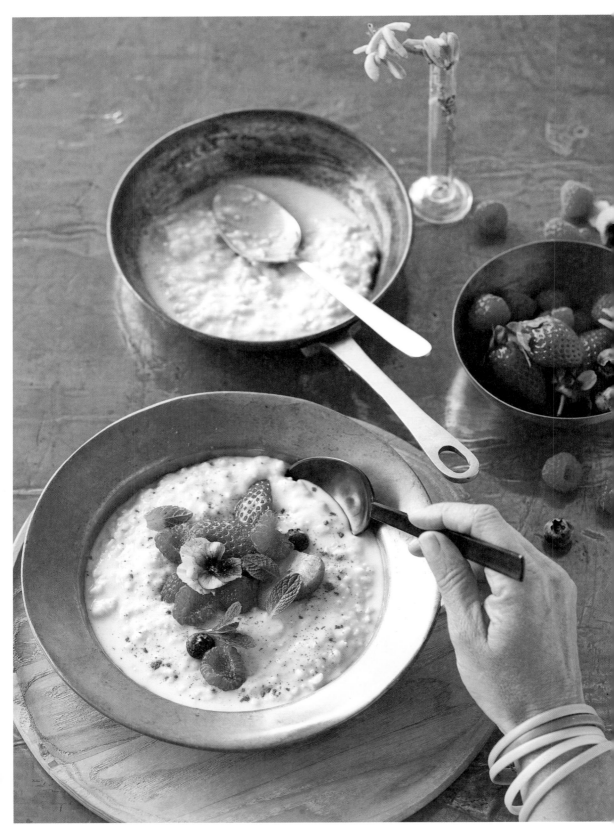

GUTMEAL
(OATMEAL WITH A GUT-HEALING TWIST)

● GF ● WF ○ DF ● VEG

SERVES 2

A big bowl of oatmeal on a cold morning is like a warm hug for your insides. Oats are one of the yummiest magical gut-healthy foods around, boosting beneficial bacteria in the gastrointestinal tract, and relieving issues such as inflammatory bowel disease, irritable bowel syndrome and constipation.

This gutmeal is such an easy way to squeeze in some gut-healing benefits first thing in the morning.

50 g (1¾ oz/½ cup) gluten-free organic rolled (porridge) oats
250 ml (9 fl oz/1 cup) filtered water
pinch of Celtic or Himalayan sea salt
pinch of ground cinnamon, plus extra for sprinkling
2 tablespoons food-grade diatomaceous earth (see page 43),
    such as my Love Your Gut Powder (optional)
125 ml (4 fl oz/½ cup) Coconut Milk (page 137)
1 handful of mixed fresh berries
mint leaves, to garnish

Combine the oats and water in a small saucepan. Bring to a simmer and cook for 12–15 minutes, or until the oats are tender, stirring regularly.

Stir in the salt, cinnamon and diatomaceous earth, if using. Mix the coconut milk through until creamy and smooth.

Serve topped with the berries and mint, and an extra sprinkling of cinnamon.

CHOCOLATE ZOATS

● GF ● WF ● DF

SERVES 1

From zoodles to pizza bases, zucchini really is the gift that keeps on giving, and is a great way to health hack your morning porridge, taking eating your greens in the morning to a whole new level. Your gut will love the fibre and vitamin C hit.

Fabulously healthy toppings include mixed seeds, hemp seeds, sliced banana, extra nut butter (melted), shredded coconut and berries. Don't mind if I do!

1 small zucchini (courgette), grated or pulsed in a food processor
50 g (1¾ oz/½ cup) gluten-free organic rolled (porridge) oats
250 ml (9 fl oz/1 cup) filtered water, or use Almond Milk (see Note, page 153) for a creamier version
pinch of Celtic sea salt
2 tablespoons raw cacao powder
pinch of ground cinnamon
1 tablespoon nut butter (optional)
2 free-range egg whites (optional, for extra protein)
liquid stevia or raw honey, to taste

Place the zucchini, oats and water or almond milk in a saucepan over medium heat. Mix together with a wooden spoon and bring to the boil. Stir in the salt, cacao powder, cinnamon and nut butter, if using.

Reduce the heat and simmer for 10–15 minutes, or until the mixture thickens; it should be like creamy oatmeal. If using the egg whites, stir them through and simmer for 1–2 minutes, or until cooked.

Stir in your sweetener of choice and serve with your favourite toppings.

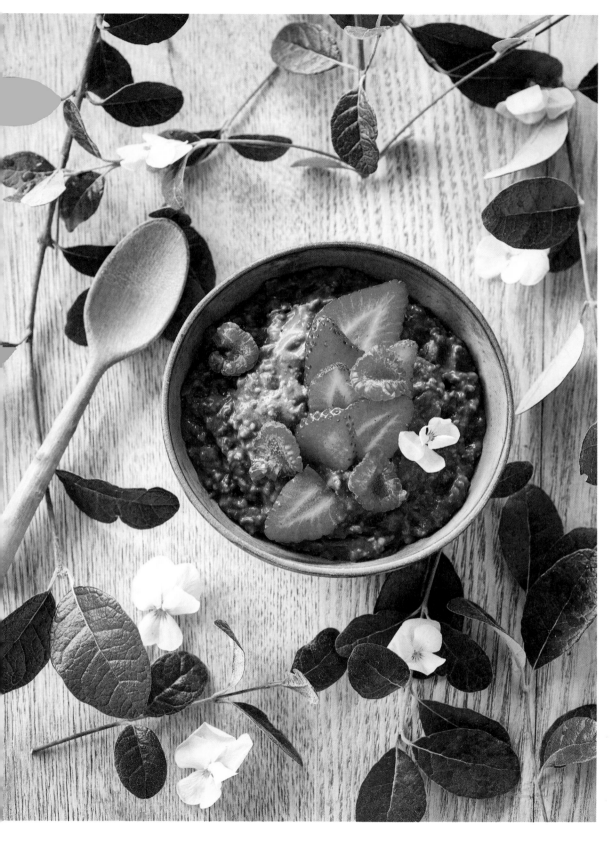

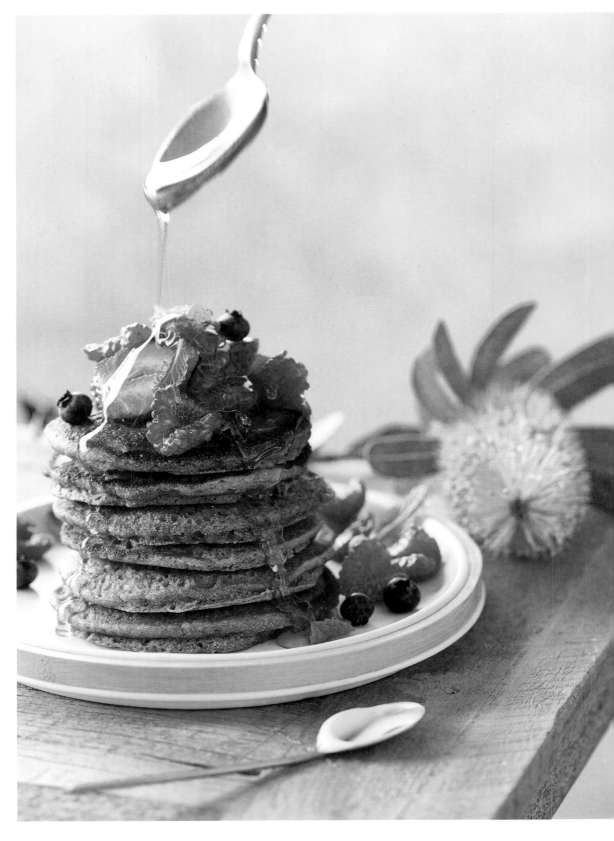

BANANA FLOUR PANCAKES

● GF ● WF ● DF

SERVES 2

A great way to feed your microbes and encourage a healthy diversity of bacteria, these tasty banana flour pancakes also deliver a hit of resistant starch to increase the production of short-chain fatty acids, which lowers the pH of the bowel, making it harder for pathogens to live there — and all while you enjoy your pancakes! Super simple to make, these pancakes will be enjoyed by adults and kids alike.

Try topping with coconut yoghurt or whipped coconut cream (page 142), fresh or fermented fruits or berries (page 268), or Mango & Ginger Kvass (page 263).

1 tablespoon extra virgin coconut oil, plus extra for greasing

PANCAKES
75 g (2$\frac{1}{2}$ oz/$\frac{1}{2}$ cup) green banana (plantain) flour
3 free-range eggs
1$\frac{1}{2}$ teaspoons baking powder (gluten- and aluminium-free)
1 teaspoon alcohol-free vanilla extract or vanilla powder
$\frac{1}{2}$ teaspoon Celtic sea salt
$\frac{1}{2}$ teaspoon ground cinnamon
1 tablespoon raw honey or rice malt syrup, or 6 drops
  of liquid stevia (optional)
60 ml (2 fl oz/$\frac{1}{4}$ cup) non-dairy milk of your choice;
  Cashew Milk (page 136) is nice

Combine all the pancake ingredients in a large mixing bowl. The batter should be thick, but pourable; add extra milk if it's too thick. Allow the batter to rest for a few minutes.

Melt the coconut oil in a frying pan over medium–high heat.

Add about 60 ml (2 fl oz/$\frac{1}{4}$ cup) of the batter to the pan. Cook on each side for about 2 minutes, or until browned. Transfer to a warm plate and keep warm while cooking the remaining batter.

Stack the pancakes high and serve warm, with your favourite toppings.

BAKED PAPAYA WITH LIME & COCONUT YOGHURT

● GF ● WF ○ DF ● VEG

SERVES 2

A zesty and refreshing source of digestive enzymes to boost gut health and start the day with a fruity twist.

1 large papaya, cut in half, seeds removed
1 teaspoon ground cinnamon
zest and juice of 1 lime
250 g (9 oz/1 cup) coconut yoghurt

Preheat the oven to 180°C (350°F). Line a baking tray with baking paper.

Place the papaya on the baking tray. Sprinkle with the cinnamon and lime zest, and drizzle with the lime juice.

Bake for about 15 minutes, or until the papaya is lightly coloured. Remove from the oven and allow to cool slightly.

Serve with the coconut yoghurt.

 NOTE: *You can add some lime slices to the baking tray to caramelise them, then squeeze the juice over the papaya just before serving.*

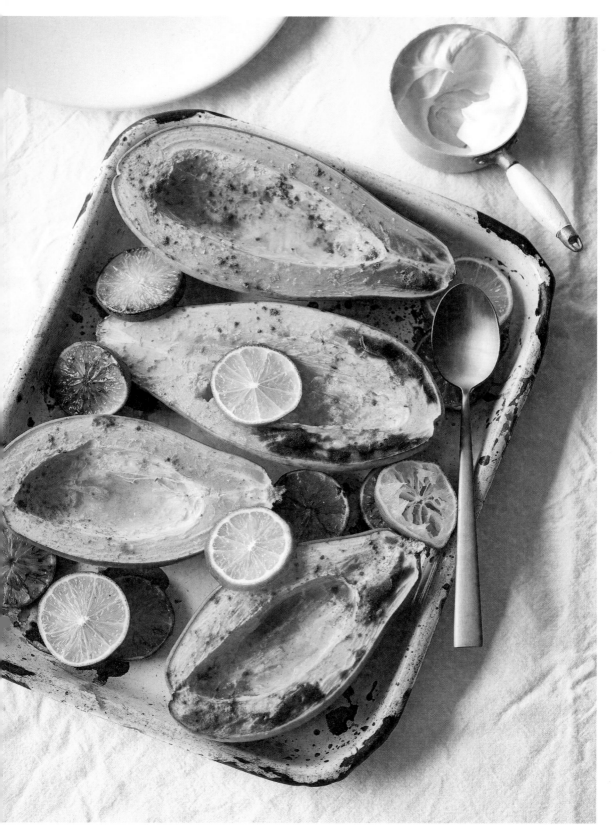

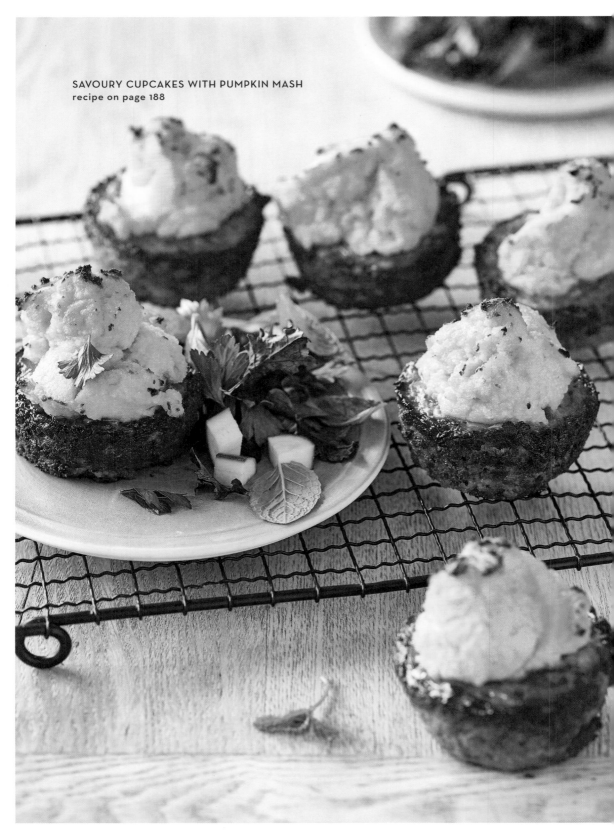

SAVOURY CUPCAKES WITH PUMPKIN MASH
recipe on page 188

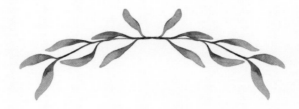

GUT GRAZERS

Graze to your gut's content with these tasty tummy-loving treats. No cooking skills required — a sense of fun and adventure is all you need to create these nutritious nibbles.

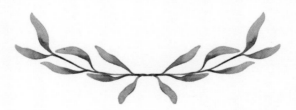

HERB-ROASTED BONE MARROW WITH GARLIC

● GF ● WF ○ DF ● SF

SERVES 2

This is a wonderful and inexpensive way to boost your gut with minerals and anti-inflammatory benefits. Bone marrow is considered a delicacy in many parts of the world, but you don't need to go to fancy restaurants to enjoy this beautiful nourishing food. Ask for marrow bones from pasture-fed animals at your local butcher or market.

Once you've eaten the marrow, you can use the bones to make a bone broth. For more about bone broths, head on over to pages 108–109.

2 garlic cloves, crushed
1 teaspoon chopped fresh rosemary, or dried rosemary
1 teaspoon chopped fresh thyme, or dried thyme
pinch of Celtic sea salt
1 tablespoon extra virgin olive oil or coconut oil
6 beef marrow bones

Preheat the oven to 200°C (400°F).

In a small bowl, mix the garlic, herbs and salt with the olive oil and a generous sprinkling of freshly ground black pepper.

Place the bones in a baking dish and cover with the herb mix. Roast for 25–30 minutes, ensuring the marrow is no longer pink, but is still tender.

Using a spoon, scoop out the marrow and enjoy.

Any leftovers can be stored in an airtight container in the fridge for up to 2 days and used to enhance broths.

SUPERCHARGED TIP

While salt may seem an insignificant ingredient, it deserves a standing ovation, but only if you choose nature's best. Salt is essential for life, but comparing the cheap 'table' variety to fine-quality salt is like comparing a billy cart to a Porsche. Table salt can overburden our elimination and detoxification systems, whereas the good stuff — Celtic sea salt and Himalayan salt — has a range of extra trace elements and minerals that shaker salt just can't compete with. Plus, you need only a smidgen to get loads of wonderful flavour.

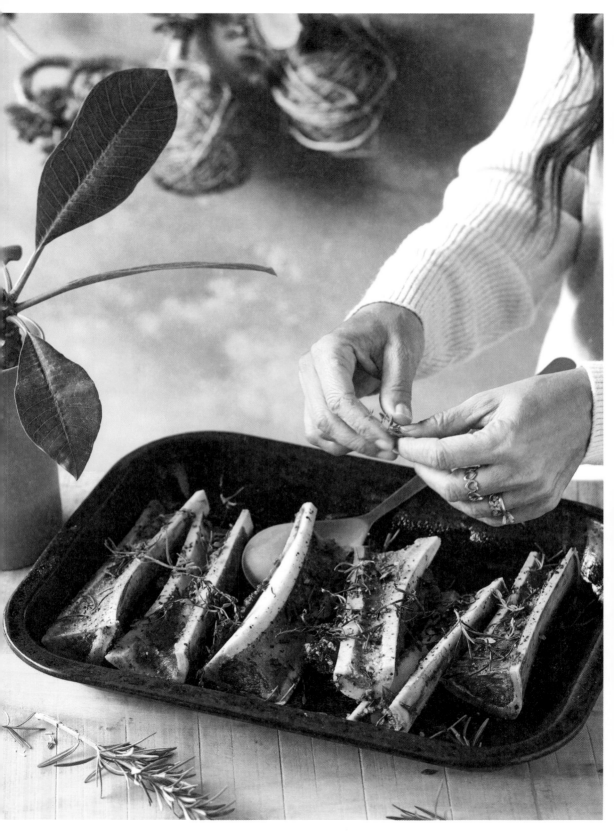

ALMOND & BUCKWHEAT CRACKERS & PÂTÉ

● GF ● WF ○ DF ● SF

MAKES ABOUT 40 CRACKERS

If you're gonna snack, you may as well graze supercharged style. Full of goodness and free of the inflammatory wheat and additives found in many store-bought varieties, these tasty little crackers are on regular rotation at our house, where they are affectionately known as 'buck cracks'. Simple and quick to make, they're a convenient snack when you feel jelly legs coming on.

To help their digestibility, serve them smeared with one of the wonderful pâtés opposite, or good fats such as avocado or the Sea Salt & Cider Vinegar Sardines on page 187.

Chicken liver pâté is loaded with vitamin E, a potent antioxidant needed for tissue repair and optimal circulation, while the salmon pâté is full of healthy fish oils to nourish the brain and provide an anti-inflammatory boost.

100 g (3½ oz/1 cup) almond meal
35 g (1¼ oz/¼ cup) buckwheat flour
½ teaspoon Celtic sea salt
100 g (3½ oz/½ cup) flaxseed (linseed) meal
1 tablespoon dried mixed herbs
1 teaspoon grated lemon zest
1 free-range egg
1½ tablespoons extra virgin olive oil

Preheat the oven to 175°C (340°F). Grease a large baking tray.

Combine the almond meal, buckwheat flour, salt, flaxseed, dried herbs and lemon zest in a bowl.

Whisk the egg in a small bowl, then slowly whisk in the olive oil. Pour the egg mixture into the dry ingredients and mix to form a dough. If it's too dry to roll out, mix in a little water.

Roll the dough out on a sheet of baking paper, to a thin rectangle measuring about 25 x 35 cm (10 x 14 inches). Place the baking tray face down over the top, then invert the two together so the dough is on top. Peel off the baking paper.

Using a sharp knife, cut the dough into 5 cm (2 inch) triangles or squares. (Alternatively, you can leave it whole and break into pieces once cooked.)

Bake for 12–15 minutes, or until crisp, turning the crackers over halfway through. Remove from the oven and leave to cool completely before serving.

The crackers will keep for up to 1 week in an airtight container in the pantry.

CHICKEN LIVER PÂTÉ

SERVES 4–6

---

3 tablespoons extra virgin olive oil
500 g (1 lb 2 oz) free-range chicken
    livers
1 onion, finely chopped, or use
    spring onion (scallion) greens
2 teaspoons grated lemon zest

½ teaspoon Celtic sea salt
1 teaspoon finely chopped
    rosemary
1 teaspoon finely chopped thyme
2 garlic cloves, crushed
generous pinch of grated nutmeg

Heat the olive oil in a frying pan over medium heat. Sauté the livers and onion for 10 minutes, or until the livers are browned, with no pink remaining.

Transfer the mixture to a food processor, add the remaining ingredients and season well with freshly ground black pepper. Process until light and smooth.

Transfer to a small dish, cover and chill in the fridge before using, to allow the flavours to blend. The pâté will keep for 2–3 days.

SALMON PÂTÉ

SERVES 2–3

---

2 tablespoons extra virgin olive oil
1 small red onion, chopped
415 g (15 oz) tin salmon
1 teaspoon grated lemon zest
2 tablespoons lemon juice

1 tablespoon chopped dill
1 tablespoon powdered gelatine
1 tablespoon chopped parsley
1 tablespoon capers, rinsed
    and drained

Heat the olive oil in a small frying pan over medium heat. Add the onion and sauté for 3–4 minutes, until softened. Set aside.

Drain the salmon, reserving about 2 tablespoons of the liquid. Remove any bones from the salmon, then place the salmon in a food processor. Add the lemon zest, lemon juice and dill and whiz until combined.

In a small saucepan, gently warm the reserved salmon liquid. Sprinkle in the gelatine and stir until dissolved, then add to the salmon mixture.

Stir in the parsley, capers and onion. Transfer to a small bowl, then cover and refrigerate for 1–2 hours, until set. The pâté will keep for 2–3 days.

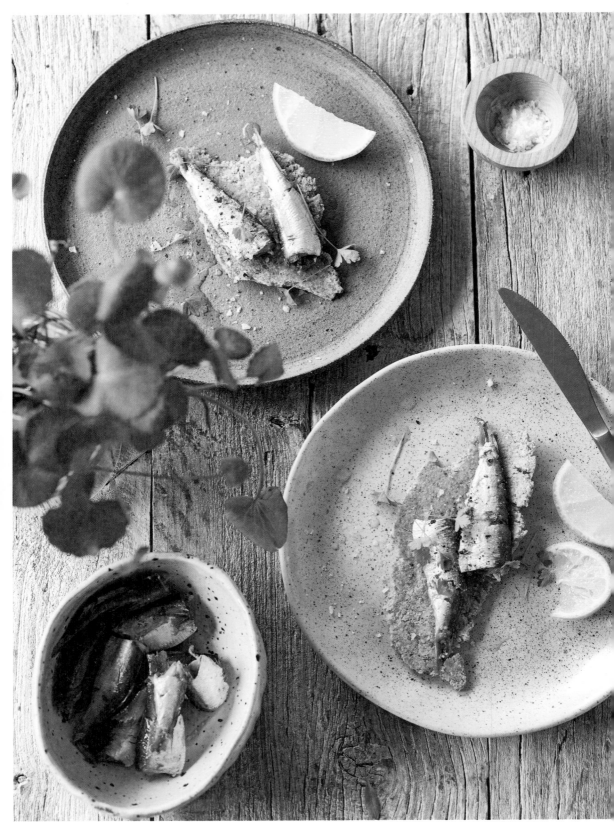

SEA SALT & CIDER VINEGAR SARDINES

● GF ● WF ○ DF ● SF

SERVES 1

Before you turn your nose up, I implore you to research some of the wondrous benefits of the mighty sardine. I've made it my mission to find ways to bring this cheap and *uber* nourishing ingredient back into the spotlight. Here's a scrumptious way to enjoy their omega-3 anti-inflammatory goodness.

110–120 g (4 oz) tin sardines in extra virgin olive oil
2 teaspoons apple cider vinegar
1 tablespoon lemon juice
pinch of Celtic sea salt
Almond & Buckwheat Crackers (page 184), to serve
herbs such as coriander (cilantro), to garnish
thin lemon wedges, to serve (optional)

Place the sardines in a bowl. Add the vinegar, lemon juice, salt and a good grind of black pepper.

Using a fork, gently mix to combine, lightly mashing the sardines if you like.

Serve immediately on crackers, garnished with herbs, and with some lemon wedges if desired.

SAVOURY CUPCAKES WITH PUMPKIN MASH

● GF ● WF ○ DF ● SF

MAKES 6 LARGE CUPCAKES

Who says cupcakes need to be sweet? These savoury ones save the day with their deliciousness. Serve warm with a drizzle of wheat-free tamari.

extra virgin coconut oil, for greasing
500 g (1 lb 2 oz) minced (ground) beef or lamb
1 onion, finely grated
3 free-range eggs
25 g (1 oz/¼ cup) almond meal
1 garlic clove, crushed
1 tablespoon mixed dried herbs of your choice, such as
    rosemary, sage, parsley, basil
2 tablespoons wheat-free tamari or coconut aminos
1 quantity warm Pumpkin & Cauli Rosemary Mash (page 209)

Preheat the oven to 180°C (350°F). Grease a large six-hole 250 ml (9 fl oz/ 1 cup) capacity cupcake tin with coconut oil.

Place the beef, onion, eggs, almond meal, garlic, herbs and tamari in a large bowl. Season with sea salt and freshly ground black pepper, then use your hands to mix and thoroughly combine.

Using your hands, scoop the mixture into six even portions and shape into balls. Press the balls into the cupcake holes.

Place the cupcake tin on a baking tray, transfer to the oven and bake for 20–25 minutes, or until the cupcakes are browned on top.

Remove the cupcakes from the oven. Using a piping (icing) bag or a spoon, pipe or dollop the warm mash on top of the cupcakes. If you like a crunchy topping, place them under a hot grill (broiler) to crisp them up a bit.

Serve warm. Leftovers will keep in an airtight container in the fridge for 2–3 days.

COLLAGEN & FLAX CHOCOLATE BARS

● GF   ● WF   ○ DF

MAKES 14

The most abundant protein in our bodies, collagen is found in our muscles, skin, bones, blood vessels and digestive tract, and is incredibly important for nourishing a leaky gut back to a healthy state. These chocolate bars are a super healthy and indulgent way to benefit from the blessing of collagen, and are also an excellent post-workout snack to help repair muscles.

You can buy collagen online or from health food stores; look for collagen derived from grass-fed sources.

3 tablespoons organic coconut butter
2 tablespoons extra virgin coconut oil
2 tablespoons flaxseeds (linseeds)
3 tablespoons powdered collagen
2 tablespoons raw cacao powder
½ teaspoon vanilla powder
pinch of Celtic sea salt
2 tablespoons rice malt syrup or raw honey,
   or sweetener of your choice

Line a very small square cake tin, loaf (bar) tin or dish with baking paper.

In a heatproof bowl set over a small saucepan of simmering water, gently melt the coconut butter and coconut oil, stirring until combined.

Place the flaxseeds, collagen, cacao powder, vanilla and salt in a food processor or high-speed blender and pulse until combined.

Add the melted oil mixture and your chosen sweetener and whiz again, adding more flaxseeds if needed; the consistency should be like a paste.

Spoon the mixture into your lined tin or dish and refrigerate for 1–2 hours, until set.

Cut into 3 x 10 cm (1¼ x 4 inch) bars to serve.

The bars will keep in an airtight container in the fridge for 4–5 days.

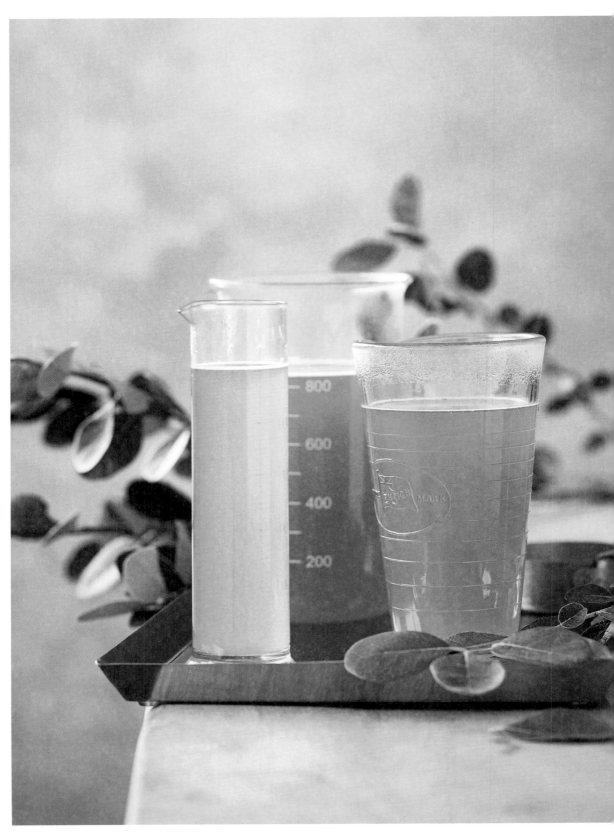

BELLY BROTHS

I like to think of bone broths as the 'green juice' of animal proteins. If you're new to them, check out my bone broth 'tutorial' on pages 108–109. I hope this chapter will inspire you to get into the kitchen and create your own wonderfully soothing, flavoursome, nourishing bone broths. They're a belly's best friend.

GUT-HEALING TURMERIC CHICKEN BROTH

● GF ● WF ○ DF ● SF

MAKES 1 LITRE (35 FL OZ/4 CUPS)

This broth uses a whole chicken, charged with the anti-inflammatory powers of turmeric and fresh ginger.

1 whole organic chicken
2 chicken feet, for extra gelatine (optional)
2 litres (68 fl oz/8 cups) filtered water
2 tablespoons apple cider vinegar
2 tablespoons lemon juice
1 large onion, chopped
3 celery stalks, chopped

2.5 cm (1 inch) knob of fresh ginger, grated
1/2 teaspoon ground turmeric, or grated fresh turmeric
a good pinch of Celtic sea salt
1 bunch of flat-leaf (Italian) parsley, about 100 g (3 1/2 oz)
2 garlic cloves, crushed

Put the chicken in a large stainless steel stockpot, along with the chicken feet, if using. Pour in the water, vinegar and lemon juice. Add the onion, celery, ginger, turmeric and salt, and season generously with freshly ground black pepper.

Bring to the boil over medium heat, skimming off any foam that rises to the top. Reduce the heat to the lowest setting, then cover and simmer for 2 hours.

Remove from the heat, remove the chicken from the pot and leave until cool enough to handle. Take the meat off the bones, reserving the bones and setting the meat aside for another use.

Return the bones to the pot and simmer over very low heat for 4–6 hours, checking now and then and adding a little more filtered water if needed.

Add the parsley and garlic and simmer for another 10 minutes.

Remove the bones with a slotted spoon, then strain the broth into airtight containers and refrigerate until the fat congeals on top.

The broth will keep in the fridge for 4–5 days, covered with a good layer of its natural fat. (Don't discard the fat — it's healthy, tasty and great for cooking with!) Alternatively, you can freeze the broth for up to 3 months.

SUPERCHARGED TIP

You can freeze all the broths in this chapter in ice-cube trays, to give convenient little portions to pop into other dishes.

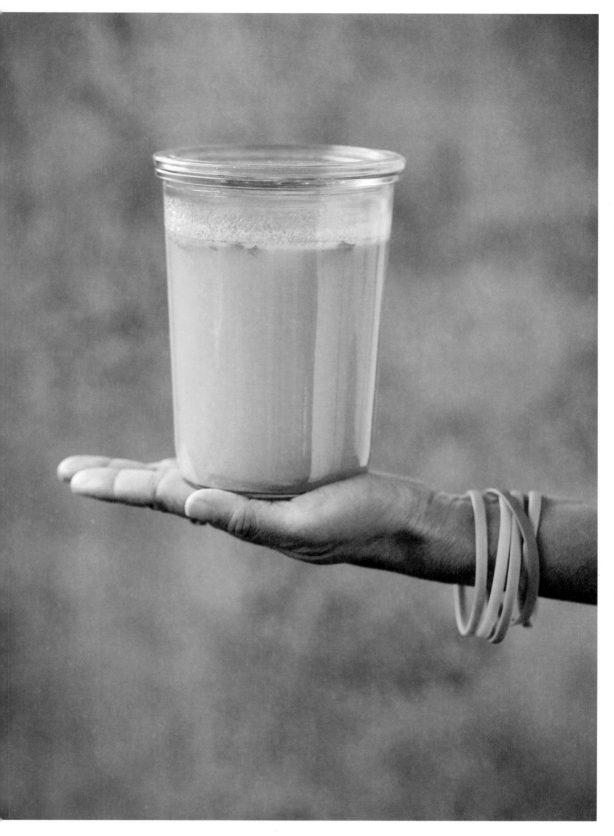

VEGETABLE BROTH

● GF ● WF ○ DF ● SF ● VEG

MAKES 1 LITRE (35 FL OZ/4 CUPS)

A vegetarian's best friend, this flavoursome, nourishing broth extracts a wealth of goodness from an array of glorious vegetables. Roasting them first enhances their sweetness and flavour.

2 large onions, skin on, quartered or thickly sliced
2 parsnips, roughly chopped
2 celery stalks, roughly chopped
1 leek, including the green bits, washed well and roughly chopped
3 garlic cloves, skin on
1 red capsicum (pepper), quartered, seeds removed
2 roma (plum) tomatoes, halved
extra virgin olive oil, for drizzling
1 small bunch of flat-leaf (Italian) parsley, about 55 g (2 oz)
4–5 thyme sprigs
2 bay leaves
1 teaspoon whole black peppercorns
80 ml (2½ fl oz/⅓ cup) apple cider vinegar
filtered water, to cover

Preheat the oven to 200°C (400°F).

Put all the vegetables in a large roasting pan and drizzle with olive oil, tossing to coat. Roast for 45 minutes, stirring often, until tender, removing any vegetables that cook more quickly.

Transfer all the vegetables to a large stockpot or flameproof casserole dish over medium heat. Add the herbs, peppercorns and vinegar, then add filtered water to cover and bring to the boil. Reduce the heat to low and simmer for 1 hour.

Leave to cool, then strain through a sieve lined with muslin (cheesecloth).

Store in an airtight container in the fridge or freezer and use as needed. The broth will keep in the fridge for 3–5 days, or in the freezer for 4 weeks.

LAMB BROTH

● GF ● WF ○ DF ● SF

MAKES 1 LITRE (35 FL OZ/4 CUPS)

Bone broths are incredible for your gut health, healing and sealing the digestive tract. If you're experiencing fatigue, bloating or even allergies, and want to show your gut some kindness, this mineral-rich broth is exactly what the doctor ordered. And there's very little effort involved — just a few simple ingredients and a good amount of long, slow simmering time.

3 tablespoons extra virgin coconut oil
1 kg (2 lb 4 oz) lamb marrow bones
2 litres (68 fl oz/8 cups) filtered water
2 carrots, roughly chopped
2 celery stalks, roughly chopped
3 garlic cloves, peeled
1 onion, peeled and quartered
1 bay leaf
2 tablespoons apple cider vinegar
generous pinch of Celtic sea salt

Preheat the oven to 200°C (400°F).

Melt the coconut oil in a large flameproof casserole dish over medium heat. Add the bones and stir to coat.

Put the lid on and transfer the casserole dish to the oven. Bake for about 30 minutes, or until the bones are browned.

Transfer the dish to the stovetop. Pour in the filtered water, add the remaining ingredients and season with freshly cracked black pepper.

Bring to the boil, then reduce the heat to the lowest possible setting and simmer for 4–6 hours, checking from time to time and adding a little more filtered water if necessary.

Leave to cool, then strain the broth into airtight containers and refrigerate until the fat congeals on top.

The broth will keep in the fridge for up to 1 week, covered with a good layer of its natural fat. (Don't discard the fat — it's healthy, tasty and great for cooking with!) Alternatively, you can freeze the broth for up to up to 3 months.

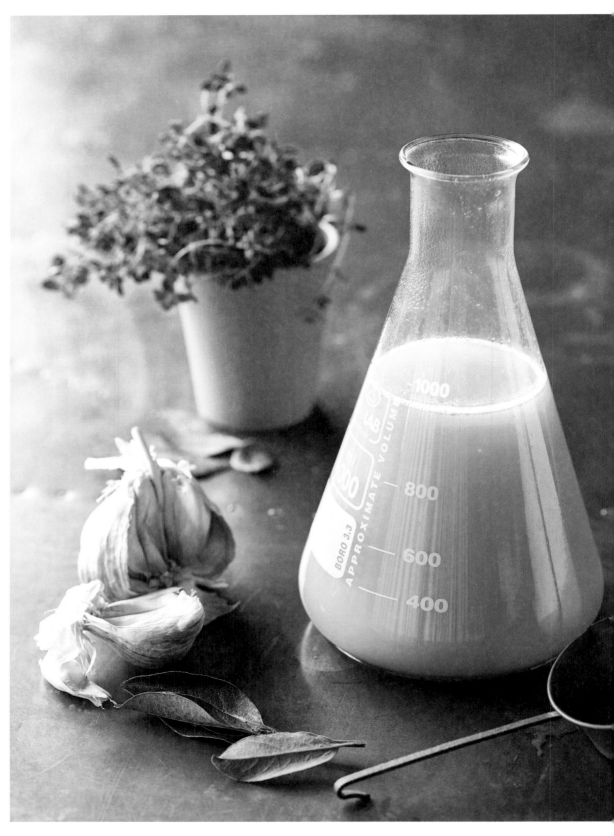

FISH & FENNEL BROTH

● GF ● WF ○ DF ● SF

MAKES 1 LITRE (35 FL OZ/4 CUPS)

Fish broths are incredibly rich in minerals and trace elements such as iodine, which is vital for thyroid function. Wonderful for autoimmune and leaky gut conditions, this broth is super tasty on its own, and makes a comforting addition to soups and stews.

2 tablespoons extra virgin olive oil or coconut oil
2 onions, cut into wedges
2 leeks, including the green bits, washed well and roughly chopped
4 celery stalks, sliced
2 carrots, roughly chopped
1 large fennel bulb, roughly chopped
4 garlic cloves, crushed
filtered water, to cover
3 fish carcasses, from non-oily fish such as barramundi,
    snapper or kingfish
4–5 thyme sprigs
2 bay leaves
1 small bunch of flat-leaf (Italian) parsley, about 55 g (2 oz)
1 teaspoon whole black peppercorns
80 ml (2½ fl oz/⅓ cup) apple cider vinegar

Warm the oil in a large flameproof casserole dish over medium heat. Add the vegetables and garlic, tossing to coat, then cover with filtered water.

Bring to the boil, then reduce the heat to the lowest possible setting and simmer for 30 minutes, checking from time to time and adding a little more filtered water if necessary.

Add the fish bones and bring to the boil, then turn heat down and skim off any foam that collects on top.

Add the herbs, peppercorns and vinegar. Cover and simmer over very low heat for another 1–2 hours.

Leave to cool slightly, then strain the broth into airtight containers. It will keep in the fridge for up to 4 days, or in the freezer for up to 3 months.

SUPERCHARGED BEEF BROTH

● GF ● WF ○ DF ● SF

MAKES 1 LITRE (35 FL OZ/4 CUPS)

Beef bones produce a wobbly, mineral-rich stock, thanks to their abundance
of gelatine. Marrow bones and knuckle bones work well for this broth.

3 tablespoons extra virgin coconut oil
1 kg (2 lb 4 oz) beef bones
2 litres (68 fl oz/8 cups) filtered water
2 carrots, roughly chopped
2 celery stalks, roughly chopped
3 garlic cloves, peeled
1 onion, peeled and quartered
1 bay leaf
2 tablespoons apple cider vinegar
a good pinch of Celtic sea salt

Preheat the oven to 200°C (400°F).

Melt the coconut oil in a large flameproof casserole dish over medium heat.
Add the bones and stir to coat.

Put the lid on and transfer the casserole dish to the oven. Bake for about
30 minutes, or until the bones are browned.

Transfer the dish to the stovetop. Pour in the filtered water, add the
remaining ingredients and season with freshly cracked black pepper.

Bring to the boil, then reduce the heat to the lowest possible setting and
simmer for 4–6 hours, checking from time to time and adding a little more
filtered water if necessary.

Leave to cool, then strain the broth into airtight containers and refrigerate
until the fat congeals on top.

The broth will keep in the fridge for up to 1 week, covered with a good layer
of its natural fat. (Don't discard the fat — it's healthy, tasty and great for cooking
with!) Alternatively, you can freeze the broth for up to 3 months.

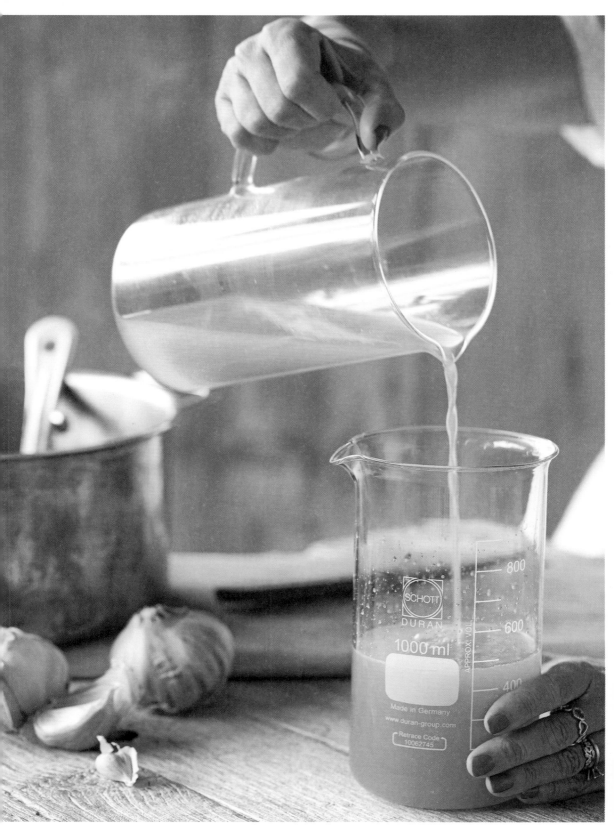

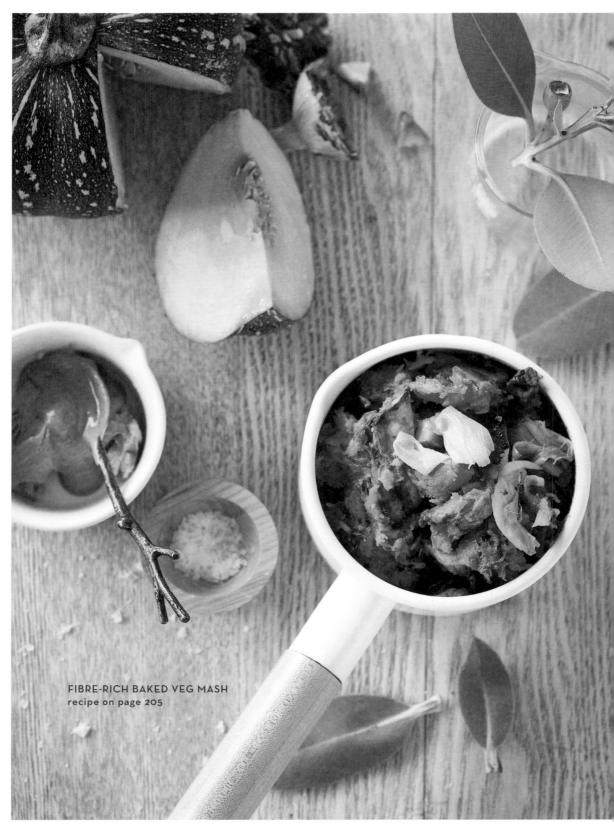

FIBRE-RICH BAKED VEG MASH
recipe on page 205

SUPER BOWLS, BAKES & MASHES

Tummy-travel to the bustling streets of India with my aromatic masala cauliflower and peas, or go all in with a tasty prebiotic tray bake, perfect for winter nights. And you heard that right — my chocolate chilli beef is no bull!

GINGER-SEARED TUNA WITH AVOCADO, PEA & MINT SMASH

● GF ● WF ○ DF ● SF

SERVES 2

Tuna is the perfect fish for loading up on selenium, with just one serve providing more than double the average adult daily requirement. Selenium is one of the minerals that is often low in people with gastrointestinal illnesses such as ulcerative colitis, and Crohn's or coeliac disease. Selenium helps modify the inflammatory response in the gut, while also providing antioxidant protection to the gut lining.

Here all the goodness of tuna is paired with a gorgeously green and super addictive — not to mention super easy! — avocado, pea and mint mash.

1 teaspoon sesame oil

2.5 cm (1 inch) knob of fresh ginger, peeled and cut into matchsticks

4 garlic cloves, thinly sliced

2 tuna steaks

1 tablespoon extra virgin olive oil, plus extra for drizzling

45 g (1½ oz/¾ cup) cooked shelled edamame beans

1 large handful of mint or coriander (cilantro) leaves, to serve

2 tablespoons sesame seeds, toasted, to serve

AVOCADO, PEA & MINT SMASH

75 g (2½ oz/½ cup) fresh peas, or thawed frozen peas

1 handful of mint leaves

finely grated zest and juice of 1 lime

1 ripe avocado, chopped

1 teaspoon apple cider vinegar

pinch of chilli flakes (optional)

Heat the sesame oil in a frying pan over medium heat. Sauté the ginger and garlic for a few minutes until golden, then remove to a small bowl.

Brush the tuna steaks with the olive oil and season with sea salt and freshly ground black pepper. Add them to the pan and fry for 2–3 minutes on each side, until cooked to your liking.

Meanwhile, to make the avocado, pea and mint smash, cook the peas until just tender, then place in a bowl, add the remaining ingredients, and roughly mash or crush with a fork. Season to taste.

Serve the tuna steaks on a bed of the avocado and pea smash, drizzled with a little olive oil, garnished with the sautéed ginger and garlic, and topped with the edamame beans, herbs and sesame seeds.

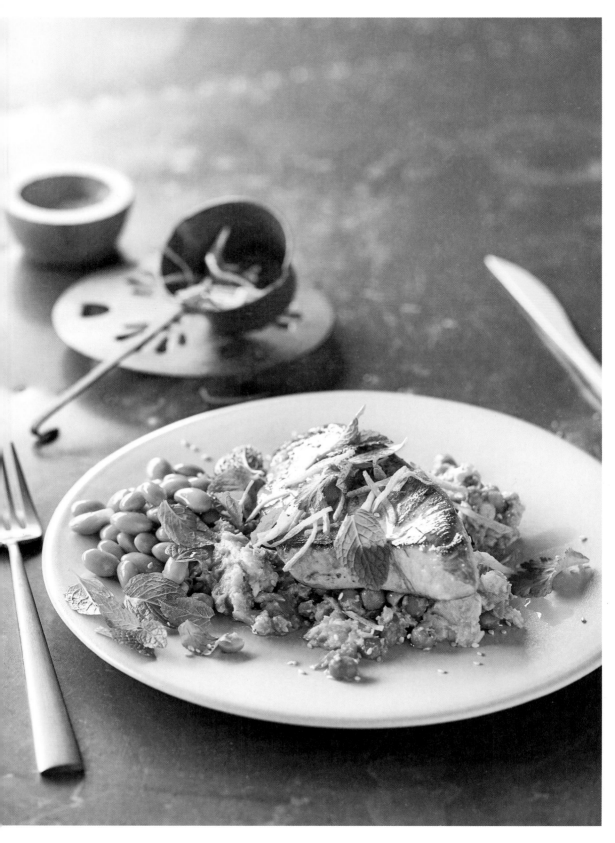

WARM GREEN BOWL

● GF ● WF ○ DF ● SF ● VEG

SERVES 3–4

Greens, greens, greens! We can all benefit from incorporating more of these detoxifying, phytonutrient-rich foods into our regular diet. They're full of chlorophyll for energy, folic acid and vitamin C, and research has also found that green vegies contain a unique sugar molecule that feeds good bacteria, allowing the good guys to take up prime real estate in our gut.

2 tablespoons extra virgin coconut oil
1 spring onion (scallion), thinly sliced
1 tablespoon finely chopped fresh ginger
1 tablespoon crushed garlic
180 g (6 oz/3 cups) broccoli florets, roughly chopped
1 large zucchini (courgette), finely diced
1 handful of snow peas (mangetout), sliced
1 teaspoon sesame oil

60 ml (2 fl oz/¼ cup) wheat-free tamari or coconut aminos
60 ml (2 fl oz/¼ cup) coconut water, or filtered water
juice of 1 lemon
1 teaspoon ground ginger
½ teaspoon ground turmeric
pinch of Himalayan or Celtic sea salt
2 tablespoons toasted sesame seeds
1–2 tablespoons Cultured Vegetables (page 264), kimchi or sauerkraut (optional, if tolerated)

In a large frying pan or wok, melt the coconut oil over medium heat until it starts to bubble slightly. Add the spring onion, fresh ginger and garlic and sauté for 2–3 minutes, or until aromatic.

Add the broccoli, zucchini and snow peas and sauté for another 5–6 minutes, or until well cooked.

In a small bowl, mix together the sesame oil, tamari, coconut water, lemon juice, ground ginger, turmeric and salt. Add to the vegetables, mix until well combined, then cook over low heat for 1–2 minutes.

Spoon into bowls. Top with the sesame seeds and fermented vegetables, if using.

FIBRE-RICH BAKED VEG MASH

● GF   ● WF   ○ DF   ● SF   ● VEG

SERVES 4

Here's a super-smooth way to get your roughage! This delicious vegie mash is suitable for vegetarians, but you can also replace the vegetable broth with the Gut-Healing Turmeric Chicken Broth from page 192.

2 large carrots
2 parsnips
½ butternut pumpkin (squash)
1 small sweet potato
1 whole leek, white part only, washed well and chopped
1 tablespoon olive oil
1 garlic clove, unpeeled
1 teaspoon lemon juice
125–250 ml (4–9 fl oz/½–1 cup) Vegetable Broth (page 194)
1 tablespoon nut butter (optional, if tolerated)

Preheat the oven to 200°C (400°F). Line a baking tray with baking paper.

Peel the carrots, parsnips, pumpkin and sweet potato, if you prefer, then roughly chop. Place in a large bowl with the leek and season with sea salt and freshly ground black pepper. Drizzle the olive oil over and rub it in with your hands, until the vegetables are well coated.

Spread the vegetables on the baking tray, add the garlic clove and bake for 35–45 minutes, or until all the vegetables are roasted and caramelised, checking now and then and removing the vegetables as they are cooked. Leave to cool slightly.

Slip the garlic out of its skin, into a high-speed blender. Add the roasted vegetables, lemon juice, 125 ml (4 fl oz/½ cup) of the broth, and the nut butter, if using. Whiz until you achieve a mash-like consistency, adding more broth if required. (Alternatively, for a coarser texture, you can mash the mixture together with a fork.)

Transfer to bowls and serve warm.

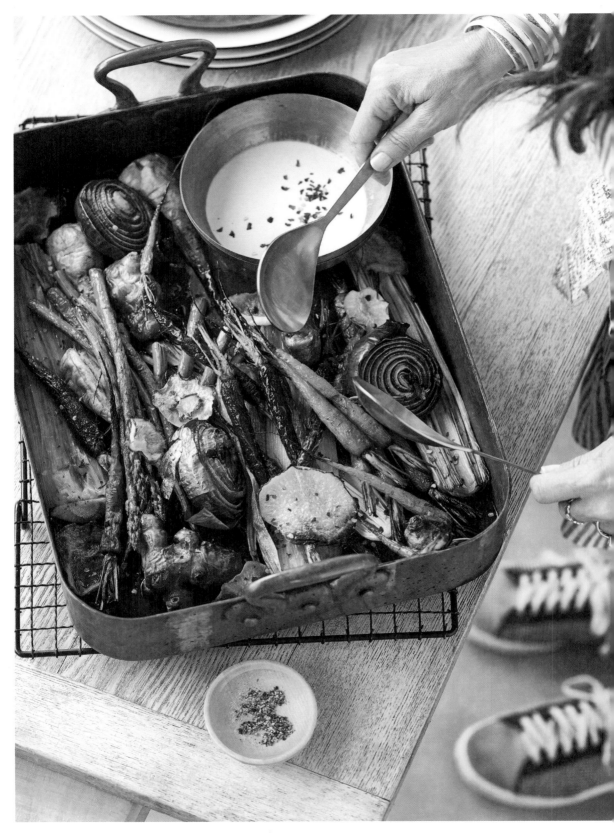

PREBIOTIC TRAY BAKE WITH TAHINI DRIZZLE

● GF ● WF ○ DF ● SF ● VEG

SERVES 4

This prebiotic bake is pimped up with a tangy garlic tahini drizzle. Roasting is a great way to cheer up any vegetable that may have been left in the fridge too long. The vegetables all cook at different speeds, so some are crunchier than others, which adds to the beauty of this dish.

200 g (7 oz) Jerusalem artichokes
½ lemon
200 g (7 oz) parsnips, peeled and quartered lengthways
300 g (10½ oz) heirloom or baby carrots, trimmed
2 leeks, white part only, washed well, cut into 2 cm (¾ inch) rounds
2 red onions, cut in half, or into thick wedges
1 jicama (Mexican yam bean), peeled and thinly sliced
12 asparagus spears, trimmed
60 ml (2 fl oz/¼ cup) extra virgin olive oil
aleppo pepper or red chilli flakes, for sprinkling

GARLIC TAHINI DRIZZLE
1 garlic clove, crushed
pinch of Celtic sea salt
3–4 tablespoons tahini (see Note, page 208)
3–4 tablespoons lemon juice,
   or more to taste
2–3 tablespoons filtered water

Preheat the oven to 200°C (400°F). Line a large roasting pan with baking paper.
   To prepare the artichokes, scrub them well, but don't peel them unless the skin seems too rough. Cut in half lengthways and immediately rub the cut surface with the cut surface of the lemon, to stop it browning.

recipe continued overleaf

recipe continued from previous page

Place all the vegetables, except the jicama and asparagus, in a single layer in the roasting pan. You don't want to crowd the vegetables, or they won't roast and crisp up, so use another lined roasting pan if necessary. Drizzle with the olive oil and rub to coat well.

Bake for 25 minutes, turning the vegetables once.

Add the jicama and asparagus and roast for a further 10 minutes, or until the asparagus is just cooked and all the vegetables are golden around the edges.

Meanwhile, to make the garlic tahini drizzle, mash the garlic and salt to a purée, using a mortar and pestle. Transfer to a bowl and whisk in the tahini. Add the lemon juice and a little bit of the water, whisking continuously, adding a little more water each time until the sauce reaches the consistency of thick cream or runny yoghurt. Taste and adjust the seasoning.

Serve the roasted vegetables with the garlic tahini drizzle.

 NOTE: *Tahini is a paste made from lightly toasted sesame seeds. It tends to separate on sitting, especially if kept in fridge. You can bring the tahini back together by leaving the jar upside down for 15 minutes, then giving it a quick stir with a clean spoon.*

PUMPKIN & CAULI ROSEMARY MASH

● GF   ● WF   ○ DF   ● SF   ● VEG

SERVES 4

For a FODMAP-friendly version, use the green part of the spring onion, and two large carrots instead of the cauliflower.

½ small jap or kent pumpkin (winter squash)
1 head of cauliflower, cut into florets
2 tablespoons coconut cream
2 teaspoons extra virgin coconut oil
1 teaspoon mustard powder
1 tablespoon chopped spring onion (scallion)
1 teaspoon fresh chopped rosemary or dried rosemary
pinch of Himalayan or Celtic sea salt
2 tablespoons nut butter (optional, if tolerated)
nutritional yeast flakes (optional, if tolerated), for sprinkling
small rosemary sprigs, to garnish

Peel the pumpkin, remove the seeds and cut into 2–3 cm (1 inch) cubes.
    Steam the pumpkin and cauliflower together for 15–20 minutes, or until the pumpkin is soft and you can poke a fork through the cauliflower florets.
    While the steamed vegetables are still hot, place them in a food processor or high-speed blender. Add the coconut cream, coconut oil, mustard powder, spring onion, rosemary, salt and nut butter, if using.
    Whiz together, stopping and scraping down the sides of the blender if necessary, until all the ingredients are well incorporated and smooth.
    Serve warm, sprinkled with nutritional yeast, if desired, and garnished with rosemary sprigs.

THAI FISH CURRY

● GF ● WF ○ DF ● SF

SERVES 4

For convenience, you can make a double batch of the curry paste, and save half for another Thai-inspired dish; it'll keep in a small airtight jar in the fridge for a week, or in the freezer for up to 3 months.

Serve this fresh, fragrant curry with cauliflower rice or your choice of side.

1 teaspoon extra virgin coconut oil

400 ml (14 fl oz) tin coconut milk

700 g (1 lb 9 oz) firm white fish, such as ling or cod, pin-boned, skin removed, cut into large pieces

100 g (3½ oz) snow peas (mangetout), topped and tailed

1 tablespoon gluten-free fish sauce

5 kaffir lime leaves, centre vein removed, thinly sliced, plus extra to garnish

2 long red chillies, seeded and sliced lengthways

THAI CURRY PASTE

2 lemongrass stems, white part only, roughly chopped (see Note)

3 garlic cloves, roughly chopped

2 red Asian shallots (see Note) or ¼ small onion, roughly chopped

1 large red chilli, roughly chopped

1 cm (½ inch) knob of fresh ginger, peeled

5 kaffir lime leaves, centre vein removed, thinly sliced

1 teaspoon grated lime zest

Using a mortar and pestle, pound all the curry paste ingredients to a smooth paste. (You can also use a food processor; you may need to add some water.)

Melt the coconut oil in a large wok or saucepan over medium heat. Add the curry paste and cook, stirring constantly, for 3–4 minutes, or until lightly golden and fragrant. Stir in the coconut milk and bring to a simmer.

Add the fish, snow peas, fish sauce and lime leaves and simmer for 3 minutes, or until the fish is just cooked; it's better to slightly undercook your fish, as it will continue to cook after you remove the wok from the heat.

Garnish with the chilli and extra lime leaves and serve immediately.

 NOTE: *With the lemongrass, you're after the tender part in the middle of each stem. Peel away and discard the tough, fibrous layers, until you're left with the white centre. Asian shallots are a red, small type of onion that can be found in most supermarkets or at your local Asian greengrocer.*

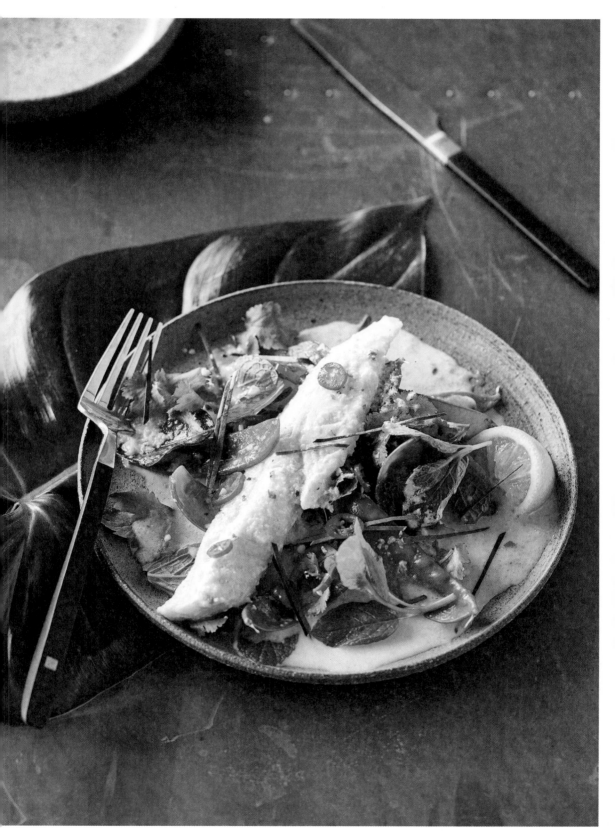

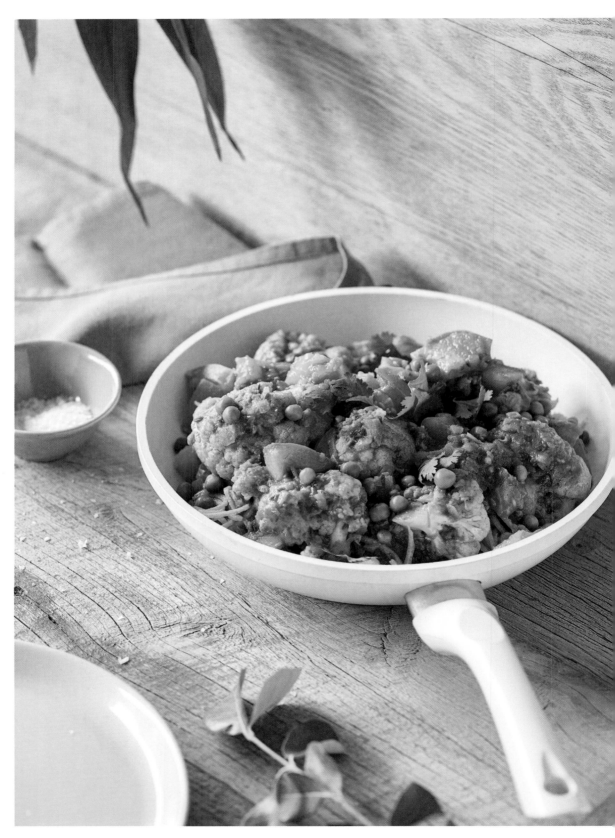

MASALA CAULIFLOWER & PEAS

● GF ● WF ○ DF ● SF ● VEG

SERVES 4

This delicious bowl takes me back to the bustling streets of India, and reminds me of the powerful nourishment and aroma of Ayurvedic spices. Cauliflower and peas are extremely comforting and easy to digest, improving your digestive 'fire', reducing inflammation and boosting immunity.

2 tablespoons extra virgin coconut oil
1 teaspoon cumin seeds
1/2 teaspoon fennel seeds
1 white onion, finely chopped
pinch of Celtic sea salt
4 garlic cloves, finely chopped
2 cm (3/4 inch) knob of fresh ginger,
    finely grated
1 kg (2 lb 4 oz) head of cauliflower,
    cut into florets
4 ripe tomatoes, chopped

2 teaspoons ground coriander
1 teaspoon ground turmeric
1 teaspoon garam masala
1/4 teaspoon chilli powder
1 teaspoon dried fenugreek leaves
    (optional)
125 ml (4 fl oz/1/2 cup) filtered water
500 g (1 lb 2 oz) fresh or frozen peas
coriander (cilantro) leaves,
    to garnish

Melt the coconut oil in a large frying pan over medium heat. Add the cumin and fennel seeds. When the seeds begin to splutter, add the onion and salt and cook for 5–6 minutes, until the onion turns golden.

Add the garlic and ginger and sauté for 2 minutes. Add the cauliflower and tomatoes and cook for 5 minutes, or until the tomatoes are soft and mushy. Stir in all the spices, along with the water, mixing well.

Cover and cook over medium heat for 10–12 minutes.

Remove the lid. Stir in the peas and cook, uncovered, for a further 5 minutes, or until the cauliflower is soft, adding a little more water if needed.

Season to taste with sea salt and freshly ground black pepper. Scatter the coriander over and serve.

CHOCOLATE CHILLI BEEF

● GF ● WF ○ DF ● SF

SERVES 4

The bitterness of cacao adds a flavourful thump to the savoury beef in this Mexican-inspired combo, while also providing a mega hit of magnesium and antioxidants. The chilli adds a hit of fire to ramp up a slow metabolism. Perfect for the cooler months.

Serve with Guacamole (page 249) and your choice of side, such as spiralised zucchini noodles.

2 tablespoons extra virgin coconut oil
1 brown onion, diced
4 garlic cloves, chopped
800 g (1 lb 12 oz) minced (ground) beef
1–2 teaspoons chilli powder, to taste
2 teaspoons ground cumin
1 teaspoon smoked paprika
1/2 teaspoon dried oregano
1/2 teaspoon dried thyme

1 teaspoon raw cacao powder (see Note)
2 tablespoons tomato paste (concentrated purée)
400 g (14 oz) tinned tomatoes
400 ml (14 fl oz) good-quality chicken or bone broth, such as the Gut-Healing Turmeric Chicken Broth on page 192
3 large carrots, grated

Melt the coconut oil in a large saucepan over medium–high heat. Add the onion and garlic and sauté for 3–4 minutes, or until softened.

Add the beef and cook for about 5 minutes, or until well browned, breaking up any lumps with the back of the spoon.

Stir in the spices and herbs and cook for 1–2 minutes, or until fragrant.

Add the cacao powder, tomato paste, tomatoes, broth and grated carrot, stirring to combine.

Bring to the boil, then reduce the heat. Cover and simmer for 1 hour, or until the mixture has thickened, stirring occasionally to prevent sticking.

Season to taste with sea salt and freshly ground black pepper and serve.

 NOTE: *Instead of cacao powder, you can use 60 g (2 1/4 oz) chopped dark chocolate (70% cacao or more). Look for one made with coconut sugar. If using cacao powder, you may need to add a tiny bit of sweetener, to taste.*

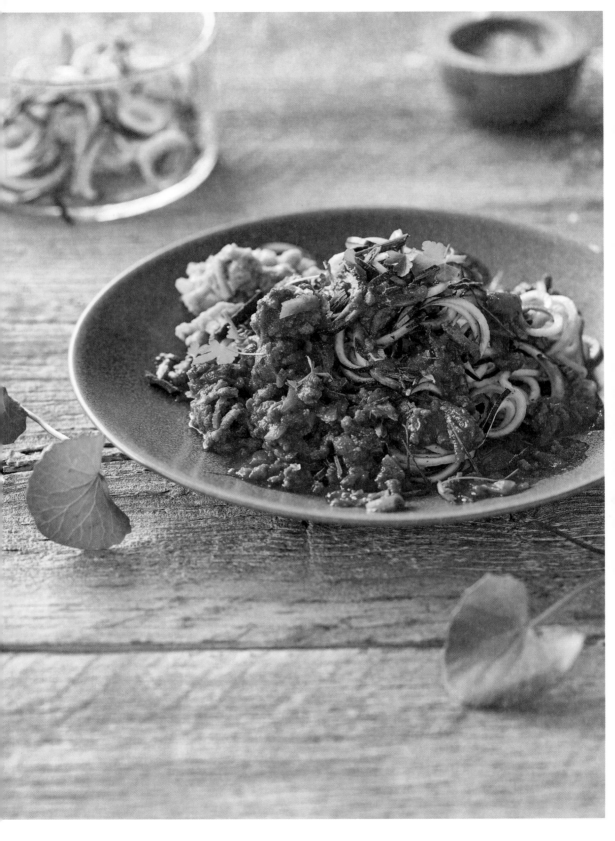

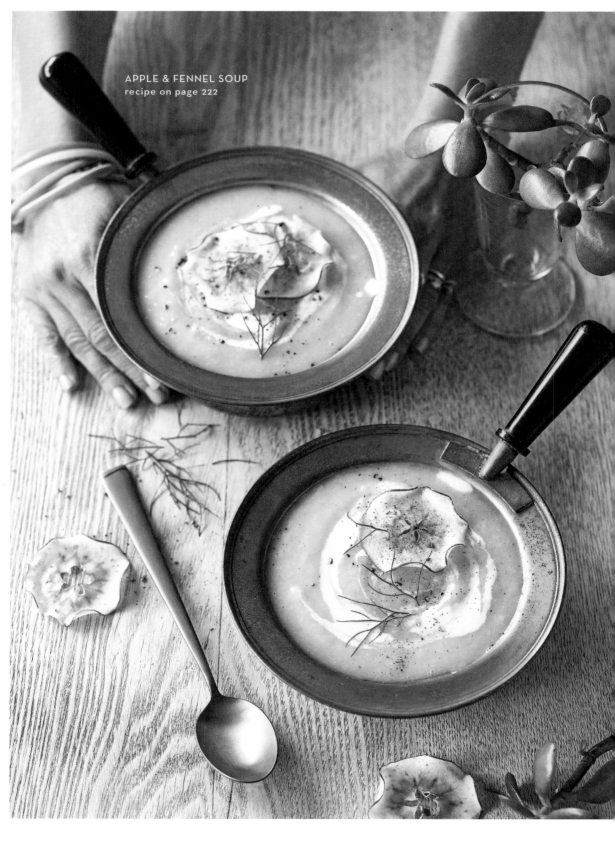

APPLE & FENNEL SOUP
recipe on page 222

SOUP IT UP

Reset the gut with digestible bowls of comfort food that come with a money-back, no-questions-asked, gut-loving guarantee. From roasted garlic bisque to sumptuous seafood chowder, you'll find all your huggable favourites here.

BEEF PHO BROTH

● GF   ● WF   ○ DF   ● SF

SERVES 4–6

This exotically flavoured broth will whisk you away to the streets of northern Vietnam, where it originated in the early 20th century and was sold at dawn and dusk by roaming street vendors shouldering mobile kitchens.

Don't be put off by the long list of ingredients, as this wonderfully fragrant broth is very simple to prepare. It also works beautifully in a slow cooker.

1 tablespoon extra virgin coconut oil
1 kg (2 lb 4 oz) beef bones — shin, knuckles, marrow and gelatinous cuts are good
6 star anise
2 cinnamon sticks
3 cardamom pods
2 teaspoons coriander seeds
2 teaspoons fennel seeds
3 whole cloves
2 litres (68 fl oz/8 cups) filtered water

2 tablespoons apple cider vinegar
1 brown onion, thinly sliced
7.5 cm (3 inch) knob of fresh ginger, peeled and chopped
1 tablespoon wheat-free tamari
500 g (1 lb 2 oz) beef sirloin, thinly sliced
3 zucchini (courgettes), spiralised
1 handful of bean sprouts
1 large handful of mixed fresh basil, mint and coriander (cilantro)
2 limes, cut into wedges or cheeks

Preheat the oven to 200°C (400°F). Melt the coconut oil in a flameproof casserole dish over medium heat. Add the bones and stir to coat. Put the lid on, transfer the dish to the oven and bake for 30 minutes, or until the bones are browned. Place the casserole dish back on the stovetop.

In a dry frying pan, toast the spices over medium heat for 2 minutes, or until fragrant. Add them to the casserole dish with the filtered water and vinegar. Season with sea salt and freshly ground black pepper. Bring to the boil, reduce the heat to the lowest setting, then simmer for 1½ hours, adding a little more filtered water from time to time if necessary.

Using tongs, carefully remove and discard the bones. Allow the broth to cool, refrigerate, then scrape off any congealed fat on top (keep it for cooking with).

Add a bit of the stock fat to a frying pan and lightly sauté the onion and ginger. Transfer the mixture to the casserole dish. Bring back to the boil, stir in the tamari and season to taste.

To serve, arrange the beef and zucchini in bowls. Pour in the boiling broth and top with the bean sprouts and herbs. Serve with lime wedges.

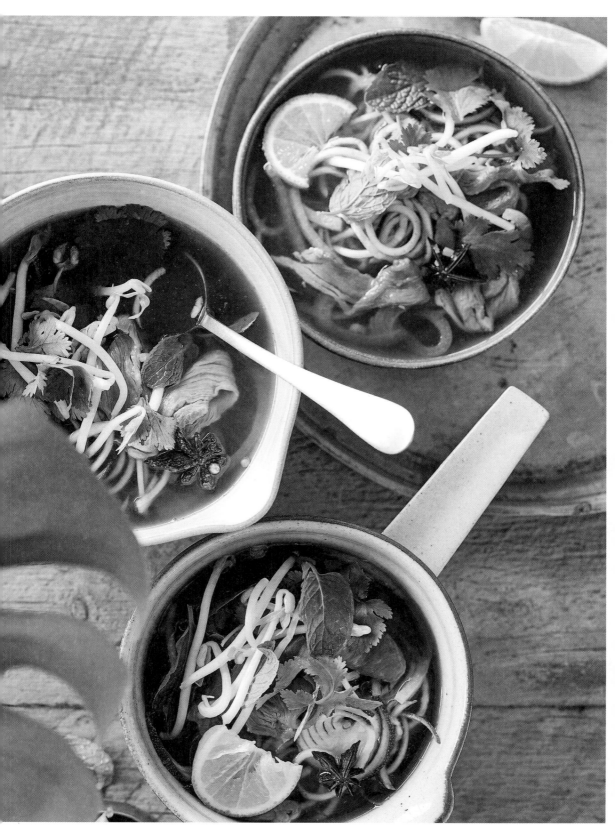

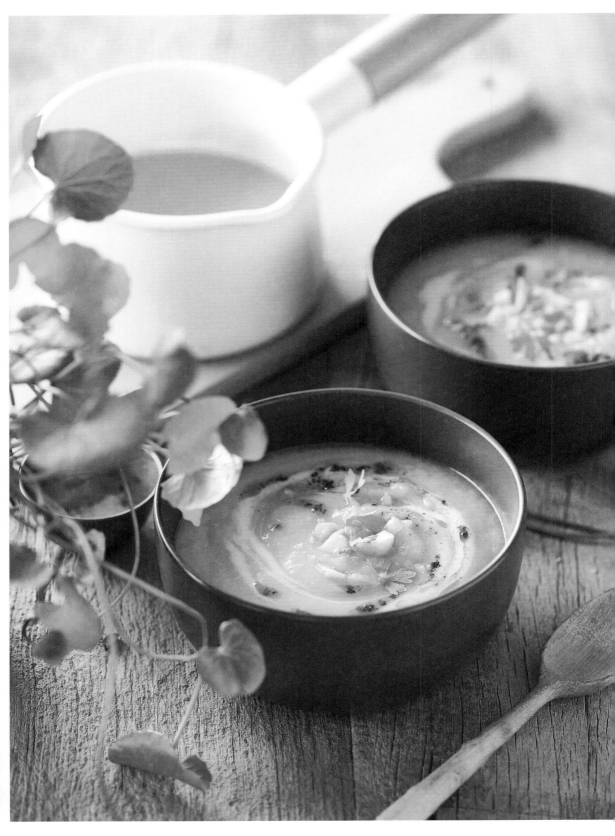

ROASTED GARLIC BISQUE

● GF ● WF ○ DF ● SF

SERVES 4

This thick, creamy, garlicky darling will provide comfort and beckon you to stop, rest and enjoy. Garlic is a wonder ingredient for rebooting your immune system, which may be compromised in cases of digestive issues or autoimmunity. The crushed macadamias add texture, but they're optional.

4 garlic bulbs, unpeeled
60 ml (2 fl oz/¼ cup) extra virgin olive or coconut oil
1 brown onion, roughly chopped
1 leek, white part only, washed well and roughly chopped
1 litre (35 fl oz/4 cups) good-quality chicken stock or bone broth, such as the Gut-Healing Turmeric Chicken Broth on page 192

3 parsnips, peeled and roughly chopped
3 free-range egg yolks
2 pinches of ground nutmeg, or to taste
100 g (3½ oz) macadamia nuts, dry-roasted and roughly chopped or crushed
2 tablespoons chopped flat-leaf (Italian) parsley, to serve

Preheat the oven to 200°C (400°F).

Cut about 5 mm (¼ inch) off the tops of the garlic bulbs to expose the cloves. Place the garlic bulbs in a small baking dish, add 1 tablespoon of the oil and toss to coat. Turn the garlic cut side up, then cover the dish tightly with foil.

Bake for 30–35 minutes, or until the garlic skins are golden brown and the cs are tender. Leave to cool, then squeeze the garlic out of the skins.

Heat the remaining olive oil in a large saucepan over medium heat. Sauté the onion and leek for 3–4 minutes, or until softened.

Add the roasted garlic, stock and parsnip. Reduce the heat to low, then cover and simmer for about 30–35 minutes, or until the vegetables are tender.

Leave to cool slightly, then purée the soup using a food processor or hand-held stick blender.

In a small bowl, whisk the egg yolks. While the soup is still warm, and with the food processor or blender still running, add the egg yolks and whiz until combined. Season to taste with the nutmeg, and sea salt and freshly ground black pepper.

If you need to warm the soup to serve, stir gently over low heat until heated through, but no longer than 1–2 minutes, or the yolks will curdle.

Ladle into bowls, top with the macadamias and parsley and serve.

APPLE & FENNEL SOUP

● GF ● WF ○ DF ● SF ● VEG (IF VEGETABLE BROTH USED)

SERVES 4

With this soup there's no such thing as pot luck. The aniseed flavour of the fennel and the apple combine perfectly on autumn nights to cosy up your insides.

2 tablespoons extra virgin olive oil
1 brown onion, peeled and diced
2 celery stalks, roughly chopped
3 garlic cloves, finely chopped
4 small fennel bulbs, with fronds
1 teaspoon dijon mustard
1 litre (35 fl oz/4 cups) good-quality chicken, vegetable or bone broth,
    such as the Gut-Healing Turmeric Chicken Broth on page 192
4 granny smith or seasonal apples, peeled and chopped
juice of 1 lemon
coconut cream or coconut yoghurt, to serve

Heat the olive oil in a large stockpot or saucepan over medium heat. Sauté the onion, celery and garlic for 3–4 minutes, or until softened.

Meanwhile, remove the fronds from the fennel and reserve for garnishing. Dice the fennel bulbs and set aside.

Add the mustard to the pan, stirring well. Stir in the stock, fennel and apple. Bring to the boil, then reduce the heat to a simmer.

Cover and cook for 30–35 minutes, or until the fennel is tender.

Leave to cool slightly, then purée the soup using a food processor or hand-held stick blender. Whisk in the lemon juice, then season to taste with sea salt and freshly ground black pepper. Gently reheat the soup, if needed.

Ladle into bowls, add a swirl of coconut cream, garnish with the reserved fennel fronds and serve.

 NOTE: *I've also garnished the soup with slices of dried apple. Simply roast some thinly sliced apple pieces in a 160°C (315°F) oven for 15–20 minutes, until dried.*

CLEANSING GREEN MINESTRONE

● GF   ● WF   ● DF   ● SF   ● VEG

SERVES 4

Soups can really help reset and gently detox the body when your digestive system is in need of a little rest. This soup has the goodness of leek and spring onion, which, like other members of the allium family, are rich in organosulfur compounds, helping your liver deal with toxins, and also reducing inflammation, while leafy greens help to move bile and break down fats in the body. So tuck in, this quick and easy minestrone is good for you — and tastes delicious too!

1 tablespoon extra virgin coconut oil
1 large leek, white part only, washed well and sliced
2 celery stalks, roughly chopped
1 litre (35 fl oz/4 cups) Vegetable Broth (page 194)
2 zucchini (courgettes), diced
1 large green capsicum (pepper), diced
100 g (3½ oz) dark leafy greens, such as kale or silverbeet (Swiss chard), chopped

250 g (9 oz) fresh peas, or thawed frozen peas
30 g (1 oz/½ cup) sliced spring onions (scallions)
1 handful of fresh herbs, such as flat-leaf (Italian) parsley, basil or coriander (cilantro)

Heat the olive oil in a deep saucepan over low heat. Sauté the leek and celery for 2–3 minutes, or until softened.

Add the broth, zucchini, capsicum and greens, stirring to combine. Bring to a gentle boil, then simmer over low heat for 10 minutes.

Stir in the peas and spring onion and simmer for another 3 minutes.

Season to taste with sea salt and freshly ground pepper, stir in the herbs and serve.

SUPERCHARGED TIP

You can serve the minestrone sprinkled with nori flakes or nutritional yeast flakes, or with a squeeze of lemon juice, or topped with a generous dollop of avocado. For a creamy version, add 170 ml (5½ fl oz/⅔ cup) Coconut Milk (page 137).

SEAFOOD CHOWDER

● GF ● WF ○ DF ● SF

SERVES 4

Say 'chow' to my creamy chowder full of delicious flavours and fibre-rich vegies. It's the perfect one-pot wonder for mid-week meals.

1 tablespoon extra virgin olive oil
2 brown onions, finely chopped
2 celery stalks, thinly sliced
1 garlic clove, crushed
400 ml (14 fl oz) tin coconut cream
500 ml (17 fl oz/2 cups) good-quality fish stock, such as the Fish & Fennel
    Broth on page 197
350 g (12 oz) sweet potato, peeled and cut into 1 cm (½ inch) cubes,
    or spiralised
150 g (5½ oz/1 cup) fresh peas, or thawed frozen peas
500 g (1 lb 2 oz) firm white fish, such as perch or cod, pin-boned,
    skin removed, and cut into large chunks
24 mussels, scrubbed well, beards removed
2 tablespoons chopped flat-leaf (Italian) parsley, to garnish

Heat the olive oil in a large saucepan over medium heat. Sauté the onion for 3 minutes, or until it starts to soften, then add the celery and garlic and cook for a further 1–2 minutes.

Stir in the coconut cream, stock and sweet potato. Bring to the boil, then reduce the heat and simmer for 20 minutes, or until the sweet potato is soft when pierced with a fork. (If using spiralised sweet potato, add for the last 5 minutes of cooking.)

Stir in the peas and fish and cook for 3 minutes, or until the fish is just opaque.

Add the mussels and cook for a further 3 minutes, or until the mussels have popped open. Discard any that remain closed.

Season to taste with sea salt and freshly ground black pepper. Serve in deep bowls, with the parsley scattered over.

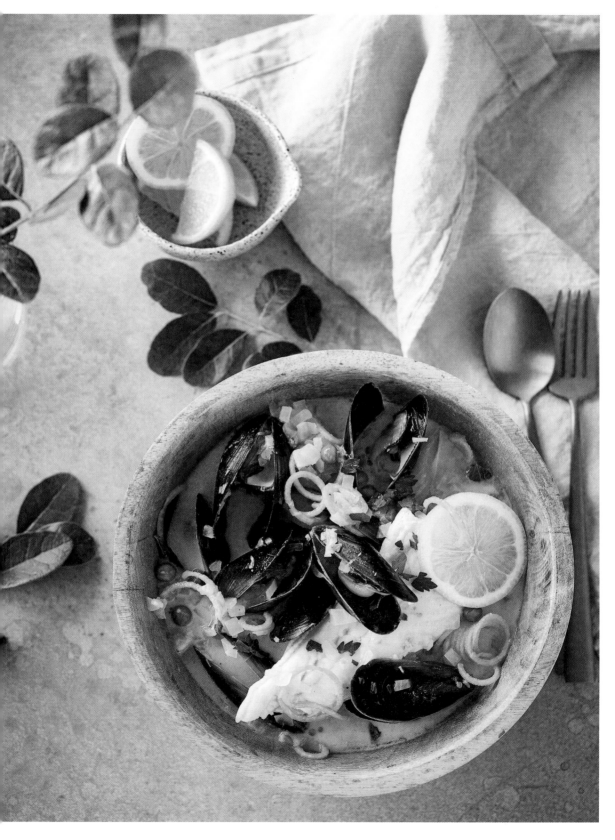

CREAMY MACADAMIA, GARLIC & PARSNIP SOUP

● GF ● WF ● DF ● SF ● VEG

SERVES 4

Macadamia nuts make a brilliantly creamy dairy-free milk, adding a dreamy smoothness and mild flavour to bring this soup together. Many studies are showing that nuts are great for feeding the gut and increasing the growth of beneficial bacteria. When blended in soups, nuts can be easier on the gut.

3 large parsnips, peeled and cut into 1 cm (½ inch) rounds
1 large onion, roughly chopped
8–10 garlic cloves, peeled
1 tablespoon extra virgin olive oil, plus extra to serve
1 litre (35 fl oz/4 cups) filtered water
155 g (5½ oz/1 cup) raw macadamia nuts, soaked in
   filtered water for at least 4 hours, then drained
1 tablespoon apple cider vinegar
2 fresh thyme sprigs, leaves picked, or 1 teaspoon
   dried thyme, plus extra to serve

Preheat the oven to 200°C (400°F). Line a baking tray with baking paper.
   Place the parsnip, onion and garlic in a bowl, drizzle with the olive oil and toss to coat.
   Spread the vegetable mixture on the baking tray and bake for 15–20 minutes, or until tender and lightly browned.
   Bring the filtered water to the boil.
   Transfer the roasted vegetables to a heatproof blender. Add the macadamias, vinegar and thyme. Season with sea salt and freshly ground pepper. Pour in half the hot filtered water and carefully blend until smooth and creamy. Gradually add the remaining filtered water.
   Ladle into serving bowls, garnish with a final drizzle of olive oil and extra thyme sprigs and serve.

THAI PRAWN, PEANUT & ZOODLE SOUP

GF WF DF SF

SERVES 2

Why order takeaway Thai when this fabulous soup is so quick to whip up at home? Prawns are a filling source of protein, while the zucchini noodles, or 'zoodles', are a more easily digestible alternative to wheat and white rice noodles, which send your blood sugars on a rollercoaster. Enjoy as a light lunch or dinner.

1 tablespoon extra virgin coconut oil
1 tablespoon green curry paste
2 tablespoons smooth peanut butter
1 thumb-sized piece of fresh ginger, peeled and cut into matchsticks
4 kaffir lime leaves
2 anchovies, chopped (optional)
400 ml (14 fl oz) tin coconut milk
200 ml (7 fl oz) good-quality fish stock, such as the Fish & Fennel Broth
   on page 197
2 tablespoons wheat-free tamari
juice of 1 lime
1 red chilli, thinly sliced
200 g (7 oz) raw prawns (shrimp), peeled and deveined
2 zucchini (courgettes), spiralised
handful of coriander (cilantro), to serve

Melt the coconut oil in a large saucepan over medium heat. Add the curry paste and peanut butter and cook, stirring, for 1 minute.

Add the ginger, lime leaves and anchovies, if using, and give a quick stir. Pour in the coconut milk and stock and bring to the boil, stirring from time to time.

Reduce the heat and simmer for about 5 minutes. Add the tamari, lime juice and chilli, then stir in the prawns and zucchini. Cook for 3–4 minutes, or until the prawns are opaque.

Serve immediately, topped with the coriander.

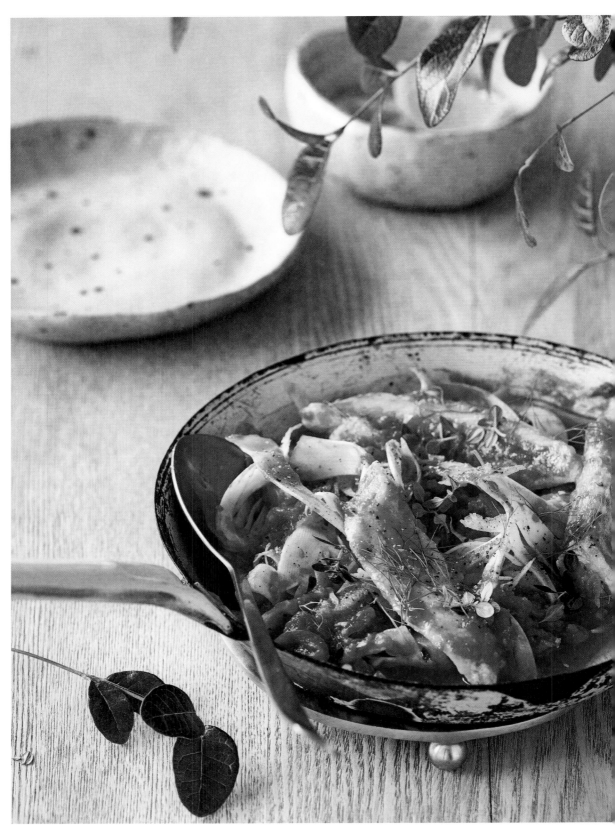

MEDITERRANEAN FISH

● GF ● WF ○ DF ● SF

SERVES 4

You don't even need to make a fish stock for this wonderful dish — the aromatics and anchovies add a great depth of flavour. Even if you don't like anchovies, use them. The dish doesn't taste like anchovies at all!

4 large garlic cloves, peeled
4 anchovy fillets
2 tablespoons extra virgin olive oil
1 large brown onion, chopped
1 celery stalk, chopped
1 fennel bulb, with fronds; dice the bulb and reserve the fronds for serving
800 g (1 lb 12 oz) tinned chopped tomatoes
2 tablespoons tomato paste (concentrated purée)

½ teaspoon sweet paprika
pinch of saffron threads (optional)
500 ml (17 fl oz/2 cups) filtered water
4 thyme sprigs, tied in a bundle with kitchen string
700 g (1 lb 9 oz) firm white fish, such as ling or cod, pin-boned, skin removed, and cut into large pieces
juice of 1 lemon

Using a mortar and pestle, mash the garlic cloves and anchovies into a paste. Set aside.

Heat the olive oil in a large saucepan over medium heat. Sauté the onion, celery and fennel for 3–4 minutes, or until softened.

Add the mashed garlic and anchovies. Cook, stirring, for about 1 minute, or until the mixture is fragrant, then add the tomatoes, tomato paste, paprika and saffron, if using.

Cook, stirring often, for 10–15 minutes, or until the tomatoes have cooked down a bit and the mixture is aromatic.

Stir in the water and thyme sprigs and bring to a simmer. Reduce the heat to low, cover partially and simmer for 30 minutes.

Add the fish, then cover and simmer for about 4 minutes, or until the fish is just cooked through.

Remove from the heat and remove the thyme sprigs. Add the lemon juice and season to taste with sea salt and freshly ground black pepper.

Serve immediately, scattered with the reserved fennel fronds.

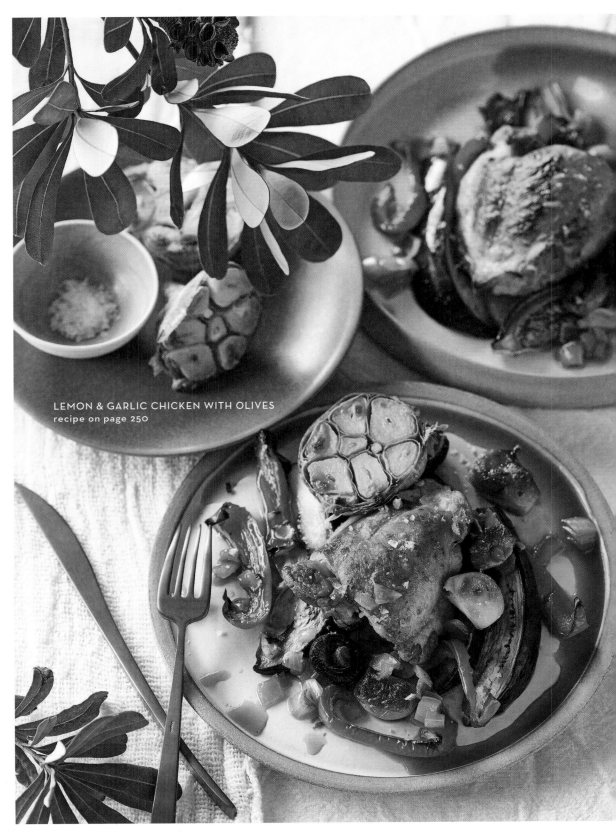

LEMON & GARLIC CHICKEN WITH OLIVES
recipe on page 250

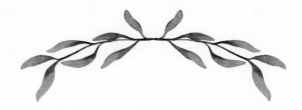

CROCKS,
CLAY POTS &
CASSEROLES

*Seal the deal with my yummy cassava and
fragrant beef curries, get saucy with a convenient
Middle Eastern meatball crockpot, and beef up
Sunday ribs by bringing together the flavours of
lemongrass and tamarind, braised low and slow.*

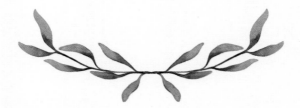

FRAGRANT BEEF CURRY

● GF ● WF ○ DF ● SF

SERVES 3–4

I love a good curry, and this slow-cooked number ticks all the boxes. The creamy coconut-based sauce is extra gut-loving thanks to its antimicrobial goodness, while the fragrant spices increase the digestive 'fire' and boost the immune system. The anti-inflammatory ginger and turmeric also help calm autoimmune reactions and stabilise blood sugars.

2 tablespoons extra virgin coconut oil
2 onions, chopped
3 garlic cloves, crushed
2.5 cm (1 inch) knob of fresh ginger, peeled and grated
1 small red chilli, chopped (optional)
4 fresh curry leaves
1/4 teaspoon chilli powder
1 tablespoon ground coriander
1/2 teaspoon ground turmeric
1 teaspoon garam masala
500 g (1 lb 2 oz) stewing beef, cut into 2 cm (3/4 inch) chunks
1 large parsnip, peeled and diced

4 tablespoons tomato paste (concentrated purée)
400 ml (14 fl oz) tin coconut milk, plus a 270 ml (9 1/2 fl oz) tin coconut milk or cream
coriander (cilantro) sprigs, to serve
toasted coconut flakes, to serve

SPICE TEMPER

1 tablespoon extra virgin coconut oil
1 teaspoon black mustard seeds
good pinch of fennel seeds
1 small onion, thinly sliced
4 fresh curry leaves

Melt the coconut oil in a heavy-based saucepan over medium heat. Sauté the onion for 3–4 minutes, or until translucent. Add the garlic, ginger, chilli and curry leaves and cook, stirring, for 2–3 minutes.

Add all the ground spices and stir for 2–3 minutes, or until the oil starts to separate and the mixture is fragrant. Add the beef and parsnip and stir well.

Stir in the tomato paste, then the first 400 ml (14 fl oz) coconut milk and bring to the boil. Reduce the heat to low and simmer for 20–30 minutes, or until the beef and parsnip are tender. Stir in the remaining coconut milk or cream, then simmer over low heat for a further 5 minutes.

Meanwhile, for the spice temper, melt the coconut oil in a small frying pan, then add the mustard and fennel seeds. When they start to pop, add the onion and curry leaves and sauté for 4–5 minutes, or until the onion is golden brown.

Just before serving, stir the tempered spice mix through the curry. Season to taste. Serve topped with coriander sprigs and coconut flakes.

CASSAVA CURRY

● GF ● WF ● DF ● SF ● VEG

SERVES 4

Cassava is a nutty-flavoured, gluten-free root used to make tapioca. It's also known as yaca and is eaten either cooked, or ground into flour and used in baking. Cassava is high in resistant starch, which helps feed your colony of good gut bugs. If you can't find it fresh, you can use frozen cassava — or make this curry with yam, pumpkin (winter squash) or sweet potato instead.

1 tablespoon extra virgin coconut oil
1 large brown onion, diced
4 cm (1½ inch) knob of fresh ginger, finely grated
4 garlic cloves, finely chopped
1 red chilli, seeded and chopped
1 teaspoon yellow mustard seeds
20 fresh curry leaves
1 bunch of coriander (cilantro), about 85 g (3 oz), stems finely chopped, leaves reserved for garnishing

1 teaspoon ground turmeric
1 tablespoon tamarind concentrate
2 x 400 ml (14 fl oz) tins coconut milk
900 g (2 lb) cassava, peeled and cut into 3 cm (1¼ inch) chunks
400 g (14 oz) tinned chickpeas (optional; see Note)
1 lime, cut into wedges

Melt the coconut oil in a heavy-based saucepan over medium heat. Sauté the onion, ginger, garlic and chilli for 3–4 minutes, or until the onion has softened.

Add the mustard seeds, curry leaves and chopped coriander stems and fry for 1–2 minutes, or until the curry leaves are crisp around the edges.

Stir in the turmeric, tamarind and coconut milk and bring to a simmer. Add the cassava and chickpeas, if using.

Reduce the heat to low, then cover and simmer for 30–35 minutes, or until the cassava is easily pierced with a fork. Season to taste with sea salt and a good pinch of freshly cracked black pepper.

Ladle into bowls and scatter with the reserved coriander leaves. Serve with the lime wedges.

 NOTE: *If using the tinned chickpeas, rinse and drain them, then soak them for 1–2 hours in fresh water for easier digestion.*

ZUCCHINI, EGGPLANT & TURMERIC STEW

● GF ○ WF ○ DF ● SF ● VEG

SERVES 4

The star of this fragrant curry is turmeric, one of nature's most powerful healers with its anti-inflammatory, antioxidant and immune-boosting properties. I add a pinch of this intoxicating, bright-yellow spice to all sorts of dishes whenever I can. Fresh turmeric, which is sweeter than ground turmeric, looks a bit like ginger, except its flesh is orange. Like ginger, fresh turmeric will keep in the freezer for a few months.

3 eggplants (aubergines), about 800 g (1 lb 12 oz) in total,
   cut into 2 cm (¾ inch) cubes
1 tablespoon ground turmeric, or finely grated fresh turmeric
2 teaspoons Celtic sea salt
4 tablespoons extra virgin coconut oil
1 large red onion, diced
3 garlic cloves, finely chopped
400 ml (14 fl oz) tin coconut cream
6–8 zucchini (courgettes), about 1 kg (2 lb 4 oz)
   in total, thickly sliced

In a large bowl, toss together the eggplant, turmeric and salt.

Melt half the coconut oil in a large frying pan over medium–high heat. Add half the eggplant and cook, stirring constantly, for about 5 minutes, or until it begins to take on colour; you may need to add more coconut oil, depending on your eggplant. Remove to a bowl.

Brown the remaining eggplant in the remaining coconut oil, adding more oil if needed, then set aside in the bowl.

Add the onion and garlic to the frying pan and sauté for 3–4 minutes, or until softened. Stir in the coconut cream, then add the zucchini and the eggplant.

Reduce the heat to low, then cover and simmer for 20 minutes, or until the zucchini and eggplant are tender.

Season with freshly ground black pepper and serve with your choice of side.

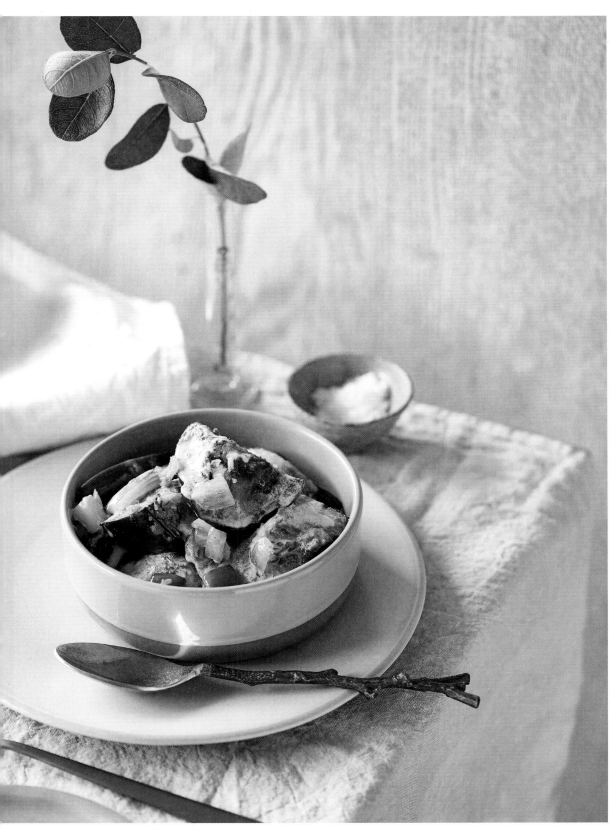

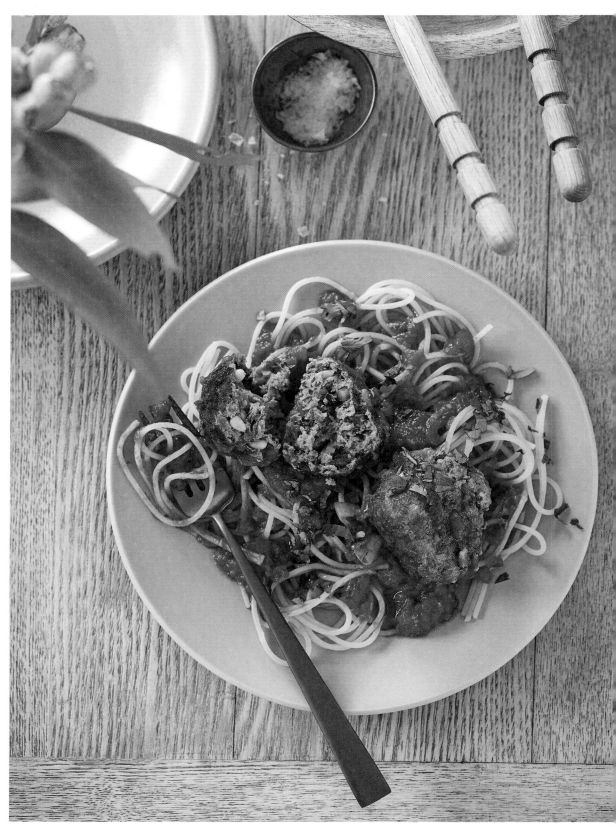

MIDDLE EASTERN MEATBALL CROCKPOT

● GF ● WF ○ DF ● SF

SERVES 4

Hearty, saucy and studded with pine nuts, these meatballs are supernaturally good. A mix of beef and pork gives a lovely texture and taste, but you could use lamb instead. Combine the simplicity of meatballs with the convenience of the crockpot, and you've got the ultimate midweek meal — one that will fill you up with nourishment, without weighing you or your wallet down.

Serve with zucchini noodles, or even a gluten-free pasta, if you've completed my 4-week Heal Your Gut program and have reintroduced it into your diet without issue (see page 71).

60 ml (2 fl oz/¼ cup) extra virgin olive oil
coriander (cilantro) leaves, to garnish

MIDDLE EASTERN MEATBALLS

400 g (14 oz) minced (ground) beef
400 g (14 oz) minced (ground) pork
2 garlic cloves, finely chopped
1 small brown onion, diced
2 eggs, lightly beaten
50 g (1¾ oz/⅓ cup) pine nuts
2 tablespoons chopped flat-leaf (Italian) parsley

2 teaspoons ground cinnamon
2 teaspoons ground allspice
2 teaspoons ground cumin
2 teaspoons freshly ground black pepper
2 teaspoons Celtic sea salt

RICH TOMATO SAUCE

2 garlic cloves, finely chopped
1 small brown onion, finely diced
2 tablespoons tomato paste (concentrated purée)
800 g (1 lb 12 oz) tinned chopped tomatoes

Place all the meatball ingredients in a large bowl. Mix together using your hands, until smoothly textured and well combined. Taking about 2 tablespoons at a time, shape the mixture into balls and set aside.

Heat half the olive oil in a large frying pan over medium–high heat. Cook the meatballs in batches, turning occasionally, for 6–7 minutes, or until lightly golden, adding more oil as needed.

Place all the tomato sauce ingredients in a slow cooker, mixing well. Add the browned meatballs, making sure they're all submerged.

Put the lid on, set the cooker to low and leave to simmer for 5–6 hours.

Serve garnished with coriander, with your choice of side.

SLOW-COOKED BRAISED LAMB WITH PUMPKIN

● GF ● WF ○ DF ● SF

SERVES 4

Lamb is one of the loveliest meats when slow-cooked, its fibres and fats breaking down into buttery tenderness. Pasture-raised lamb contains valuable amounts of conjugated linoleic acid, a health-supportive fatty acid that has been shown to promote fat loss — so it's worth buying organically raised, 100 per cent grass-fed lamb wherever possible. Enjoy its benefits in this super comforting casserole.

60 ml (2 fl oz/¼ cup) extra virgin olive oil
600 g (1 lb 5 oz) boneless lamb shoulder, cut into 3 cm (1¼ inch) chunks
2 brown onions, roughly chopped
3 celery stalks, roughly chopped
4 garlic cloves, finely chopped
1 rosemary sprig
1 teaspoon ground cumin
1 teaspoon smoked paprika

1 teaspoon ground coriander
1 teaspoon ground turmeric
1 teaspoon ground cinnamon
1 teaspoon ground sumac
750 ml (26 fl oz/3 cups) good-quality chicken stock or bone broth, such as the Gut-Healing Turmeric Chicken Broth on page 192
600 g (1 lb 5 oz) butternut pumpkin (squash), peeled and cut into 5 cm (2 inch) chunks

Preheat the oven to 160°C (315°F).

Heat half the olive oil in a flameproof casserole dish over medium–high heat.

Season the lamb with sea salt and freshly ground black pepper. Working in batches to prevent the lamb stewing, cook the lamb, turning occasionally, for about 3–4 minutes, or until browned. Remove to a plate.

Heat the remaining oil in the casserole dish and sauté the onion, celery and garlic for 3–4 minutes, or until softened.

Add the rosemary and spices and stir for about 1 minute, or until fragrant.

Pour in the stock, then return the lamb to the dish, together with the pumpkin. Make sure the lamb and pumpkin are partially submerged, adding more stock or a little filtered water if necessary.

Bring to a simmer, then put the lid on and transfer to the oven. Cook for about 2½ hours, or until the lamb easily pulls apart when pierced with a fork.

Serve with your favourite accompaniment.

GREEN BEAN CASSEROLE WITH MUSHROOMS & THYME

● GF   ● WF   ○ DF   ● SF   ● VEG

SERVES 4

Lift the lid on a 30-minute make-ahead meal that's good for the belly and perfect for those 'meatless Mondays'.

2 tablespoons extra virgin coconut oil
1 brown onion, sliced lengthways
500 g (1 lb 2 oz) mixed mushrooms, sliced
5 garlic cloves, finely chopped
1 teaspoon dried thyme or rosemary, or 1 tablespoon fresh
    thyme or rosemary leaves
250 ml (9 fl oz/1 cup) Vegetable Broth (page 194)
450 g (1 lb) green beans, trimmed and halved

Preheat the oven to 180°C (350°F).

Melt the coconut oil in a flameproof casserole dish over medium–high heat. Sauté the onion for 3–4 minutes, or until softened.

Add the mushrooms and cook for 5–6 minutes, stirring occasionally, until the mushrooms begin to give up some of their liquid.

Add the garlic and herbs and cook for a further 1–2 minutes.

Stir in the stock, and add the beans. Bring to a simmer, then put the lid on and transfer to the oven.

Cook for 25–30 minutes, or until the beans are tender.

Season to taste with sea salt and freshly ground black pepper and serve with your favourite accompaniment.

SUNDAY BRAISED BEEF RIBS WITH LEMONGRASS & TAMARIND

● GF   ● WF   ○ DF   ● SF

SERVES 4

A Sunday roast has been a ritual throughout the centuries, but in this busy day and age we sometimes forget how important and special the slow enjoyment of ritual meals can be. So, bring back the Sunday feast with this lovely braised beef. Sit around the table with loved ones and enjoy the savoury aromas with gratitude for your life, health and relationships.

1 tablespoon extra virgin olive oil
2 kg (4 lb 8 oz) beef short ribs
2 red onions, finely diced
4 cm (1½ inch) knob of fresh ginger, finely grated
8 garlic cloves, roughly chopped
2 lemongrass stems, white part only, roughly chopped
2 coriander (cilantro) roots, scraped and finely chopped
3 whole star anise
1 cinnamon stick

3 tablespoons raw honey
150 g (3½ oz/½ cup) tamarind purée
80 ml (2½ fl oz/⅓ cup) wheat-free tamari
750 ml–1 litre (26–35 fl oz/3–4 cups) good-quality chicken stock or bone broth, such as the Gut-Healing Turmeric Chicken Broth on page 192
coriander (cilantro) leaves, to garnish

Preheat the oven to 150°C (300°F).

Heat the olive oil in a large frying pan over medium–high heat. Working in batches if necessary, cook the ribs, turning occasionally, for 3–5 minutes, or until browned. Transfer to a deep roasting pan that will fit them all snugly in a single layer.

In the same frying pan, sauté the onion, ginger, garlic, lemongrass and coriander roots for 3–4 minutes, or until the onion has softened, then add the mixture to the ribs in the roasting pan, distributing it evenly. Add the star anise and cinnamon stick.

Drizzle the honey, tamarind and tamari over the ribs, then pour in the stock. Cover tightly with a sheet of baking paper, then a sheet of foil.

Transfer to the oven and roast for 2½–3 hours, or until the meat on the ribs is very tender. Garnish with coriander and serve with your choice of side.

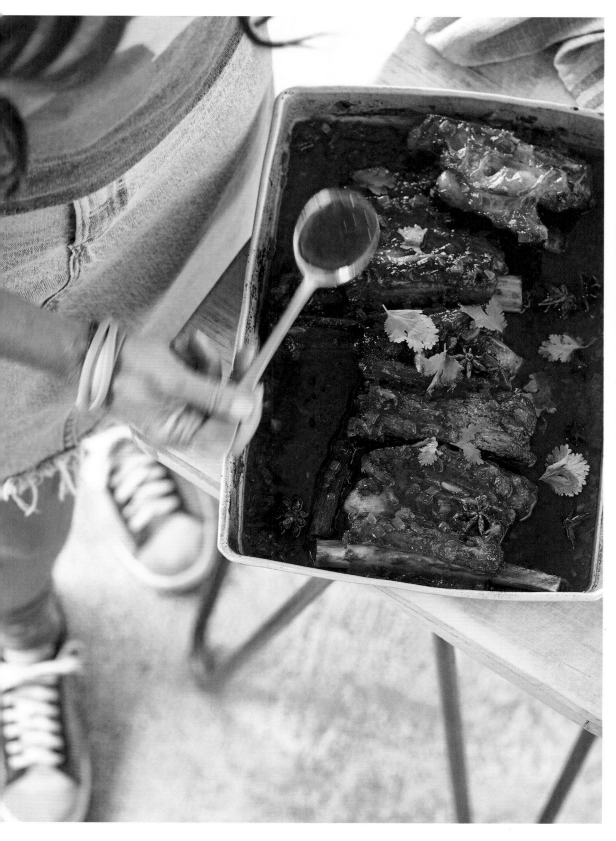

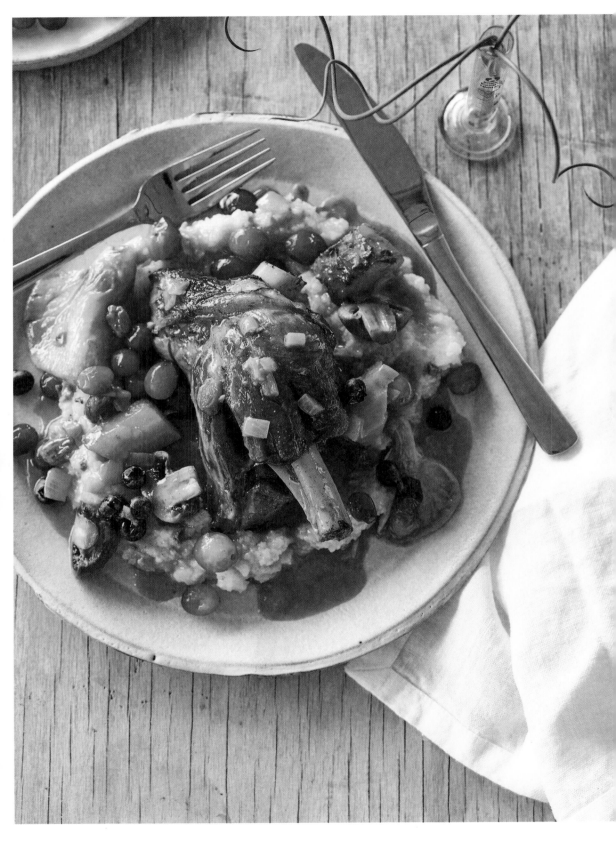

SLOW-COOKER LAMB SHANKS

● GF ● WF ○ DF ● SF

SERVES 4

A beautiful mixture of aromatic spices infuses the most delicious flavour into every mouthful of these succulent lamb shanks. Just brown the shanks and place all the ingredients in the slow cooker mid-morning and by evening you'll have an intensely flavoursome and fulfilling meal, the slow-cooked meat just falling off the bone. Instead of dried blueberries and cranberries, you could use dates or raw honey for a touch of sweetness.

Cauliflower or celeriac mash partner these shanks perfectly.

2 tablespoons extra virgin olive oil
4 lamb shanks
100 g (3½ oz) mushrooms, chopped
1 carrot, diced
1 celery stalk, diced
1 onion, diced
2 garlic cloves, crushed
2 tablespoons mixed ground spices such as cardamom,
    cinnamon, nutmeg, paprika, turmeric, coriander,
    cumin and ginger
1 teaspoon Celtic sea salt
3 tablespoons dried cranberries or blueberries (see Note)
250 ml (9 fl oz/1 cup) good-quality beef or chicken stock,
    such as the Gut-Healing Turmeric Chicken Broth on page 192
2 tablespoons lemon juice
2 tablespoons apple cider vinegar
chopped parsley, to garnish (optional)

Heat half the olive oil in a large frying pan over medium–high heat. Working in batches if necessary, cook the shanks, turning occasionally, for 3–5 minutes, or until browned all over. Transfer to a slow cooker.

recipe continued overleaf

recipe continued from previous page

Heat the remaining oil in the same pan and sauté the mushrooms, carrot, celery and onion for 3 minutes, or until softened. Stir in the garlic, ground spices and salt, cook for 1–2 minutes, then add the mixture to the slow cooker.

Add the dried berries, pour in the stock, lemon juice and vinegar, and add a few good grinds of black pepper.

Put the lid on, set the cooker to low and leave to simmer for 8 hours.

Transfer the shanks to a warmed wide serving bowl and spoon the sauce over the top. Garnish with parsley, if using, and serve with your choice of accompaniments.

 NOTE: *If you don't have dried berries, you can add fresh berries near the end of the cooking time. The shanks can also be cooked in a 100°C (200°F) oven in an ovenproof dish with a tight-fitting lid for 6 hours.*

FILIPINO-STYLE CHICKEN, MUSHROOM & LEEK ADOBO

● GF ● WF ○ DF ● SF

SERVES 4

The key to this dish is getting the right balance of sweetness, saltiness and acidity. Cooking softens the sharpness of the vinegar, while aromatics such as star anise and bay leaves build the complexity of the broth. Apple cider vinegar is full of enzymes and potassium, to aid digestion, and is great for the immune system.

1 tablespoon extra virgin coconut oil
4 chicken Marylands (leg quarters), about 1.25 kg (2 lb 12 oz) in total, skin on
8 garlic cloves, crushed
2 cm (3/4 inch) knob of fresh ginger, grated
250 g (9 oz) mushrooms, roughly sliced
2 leeks, white part only, washed well and thinly sliced, or 4 spring onions (scallions), chopped

1 star anise
4 dried bay leaves
1 dried red chilli, whole
250 ml (9 fl oz/1 cup) apple cider vinegar
75 ml (2 1/2 fl oz) wheat-free tamari
175 ml (5 1/2 fl oz) quality chicken stock or bone broth, such as the Gut-Healing Turmeric Chicken Broth on page 192
1 long red chilli, seeded and thinly sliced

Melt the coconut oil in a large heavy-based saucepan over medium–high heat.

Season the chicken with sea salt and freshly ground black pepper. Working in batches if necessary, fry the chicken, turning frequently, for 6–8 minutes, or until browned on all sides.

Add the garlic and ginger and cook for a further 1–2 minutes, or until lightly golden.

Stir in the mushrooms, leek, star anise, bay leaves, whole dried chilli, vinegar, tamari and stock.

Bring to the boil, then reduce the heat to low. Cover and cook for 1 hour, or until the chicken is tender and falling off the bone.

Sprinkle with the sliced fresh chilli, and serve with cauliflower rice or your choice of accompaniment.

BUTTER CHICKEN CLAY POT

● GF ● WF ○ DF ● SF

SERVES 4

Everything just tastes better in a clay pot — even butter chicken! This version will help give your Friday-night curry a gut-friendly upgrade.

2 tablespoons extra virgin olive oil
1 large brown onion, diced
4 garlic cloves, crushed
3 cm (1¼ inch) knob of fresh ginger, grated
2 teaspoons garam masala
1 teaspoon ground cumin
½ teaspoon ground coriander
½ teaspoon ground cinnamon
½ teaspoon ground turmeric
½ teaspoon chilli powder
1 teaspoon Celtic sea salt

750 g (1 lb 10 oz) boneless, skinless chicken thighs, halved or cut into pieces
1 bay leaf
400 ml (14 fl oz) tomato passata (puréed tomatoes)
250 ml (9 fl oz/1 cup) coconut cream
100 g (1 lb 10 oz) roasted unsalted cashews, crushed or finely chopped
2 tablespoons lemon juice
coriander (cilantro) leaves, to serve

Heat the olive oil in a large clay pot or heavy-based saucepan over medium heat. Sauté the onion for 3–4 minutes, or until softened. Add the garlic and ginger and sauté for a further minute.

Stir in the ground spices and salt and sauté for 2 minutes, or until fragrant.

Add the chicken and cook, stirring frequently, for about 5 minutes, before adding the bay leaf, passata, coconut cream and cashews.

Reduce the heat to low and simmer, uncovered, for 20–25 minutes, or until the chicken is cooked through.

Stir in the lemon juice, scatter with coriander and serve with cauliflower rice or your choice of accompaniment.

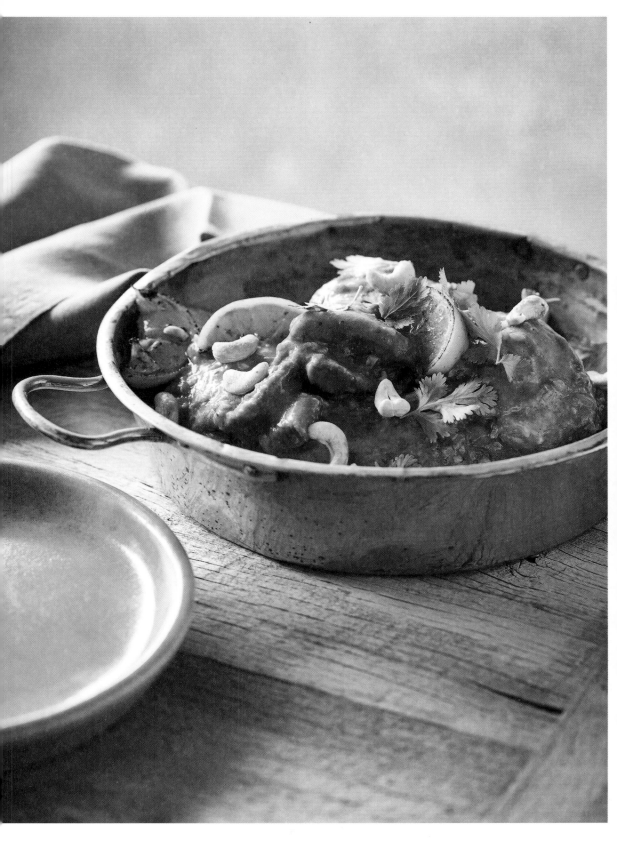

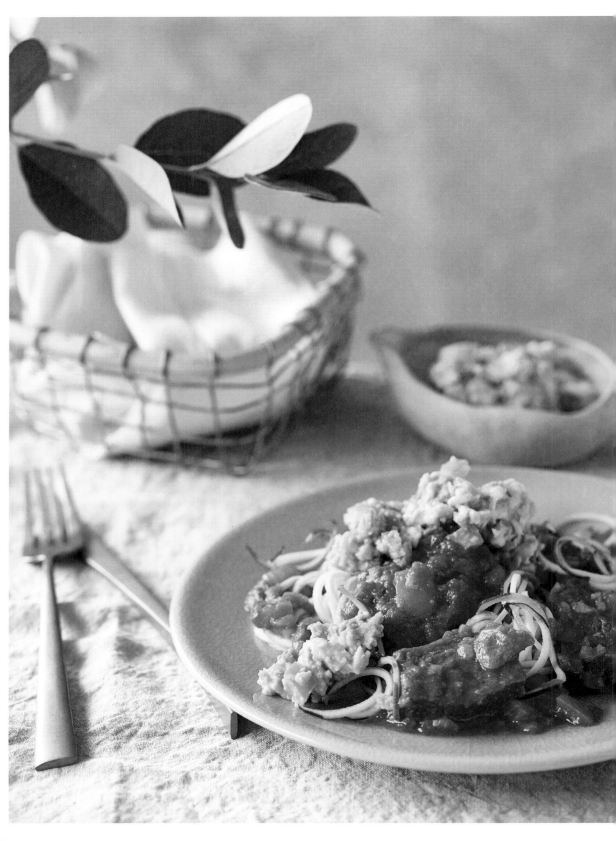

TACO BEEF STEW WITH GUACAMOLE

● GF ● WF ○ DF ● SF

SERVES 4

Mexican is one of my favourite cuisines; its exotic flavours send me into somewhat of a fiesta. Loaded with vitamins B3, B6 and B12, as well as zinc, selenium and iron, beef is also an excellent source of blood- and muscle-nourishing protein. Serve with zucchini noodles or cauliflower rice.

1 tablespoon extra virgin coconut oil
2 red onions, diced
1 capsicum (pepper), diced
4 garlic cloves, finely chopped
2 teaspoons ground cumin
1 teaspoon smoked paprika
1 teaspoon ground coriander
1/2 teaspoon ground chilli
700 g (1 lb 9 oz) stewing beef, such as chuck, rump or shin, cut into 3 cm (1 1/4 inch) chunks
1 tablespoon tomato paste (concentrated purée)

400 g (14 oz) tinned diced tomatoes
500 ml (17 fl oz/2 cups) good-quality beef or chicken stock, such as the Gut-Healing Turmeric Chicken Broth on page 192

GUACAMOLE

2 ripe avocados
1/2 teaspoon ground cumin
1 garlic clove, crushed or finely grated
2 tomatoes, seeded and diced
1 tablespoon lime juice

Preheat the oven to 160°C (315°F).

Melt the coconut oil in a large flameproof casserole dish over medium–high heat. Sauté the onion, capsicum and garlic for 3–4 minutes, or until softened.

Stir in the spices and beef and cook, stirring, for 5–7 minutes, or until the beef is browned on the outside and thoroughly coated in the spices. Stir in the tomato paste, tomatoes and stock.

Put the lid on, transfer to the oven and cook for 1 1/2 hours, or until the beef is tender and pulls apart easily with a fork. The time will vary depending on the cut of meat you're using.

To make the guacamole, scoop the flesh from the avocados into a large bowl. Sprinkle with the cumin, add the remaining ingredients and roughly mash together using a fork. Season to taste with sea salt and freshly ground black pepper.

Serve the stew topped with the guacamole, with your choice of accompaniment.

LEMON & GARLIC CHICKEN WITH OLIVES

● GF ● WF ○ DF ● SF

SERVES 4

Here's a gut-loving lemon and garlic bake that's effortless to make and suitable for the whole family to enjoy.

4 chicken thighs, on the bone, with the skin on,
    about 900 g (2 lb) in total
1 garlic bulb, cut in half
1 lemon, cut into wedges or thick slices
200 g (7 oz) black or green olives, or a mix
1/4 teaspoon chilli flakes
1/2 teaspoon fennel seeds
a few rosemary sprigs
1 tablespoon extra virgin olive oil
150 ml (5 fl oz) good-quality chicken broth or bone stock,
    such as the Gut-Healing Turmeric Chicken Broth on page 192

Preheat the oven to 180°C (350°F).
    Season the chicken thighs with sea salt and freshly ground pepper. Place, skin side up, in a single layer in a baking dish that will fit them quite snugly. Arrange the garlic bulb and lemon wedges around, along with the olives.
    Sprinkle with the chilli flakes, fennel seeds and rosemary. Drizzle with the olive oil and pour in the stock.
    Cover the dish with foil, transfer to the oven and bake for 20 minutes.
    Remove the foil and roast for a further 20–25 minutes, or until the skin is golden.
    Serve with your choice of accompaniment.

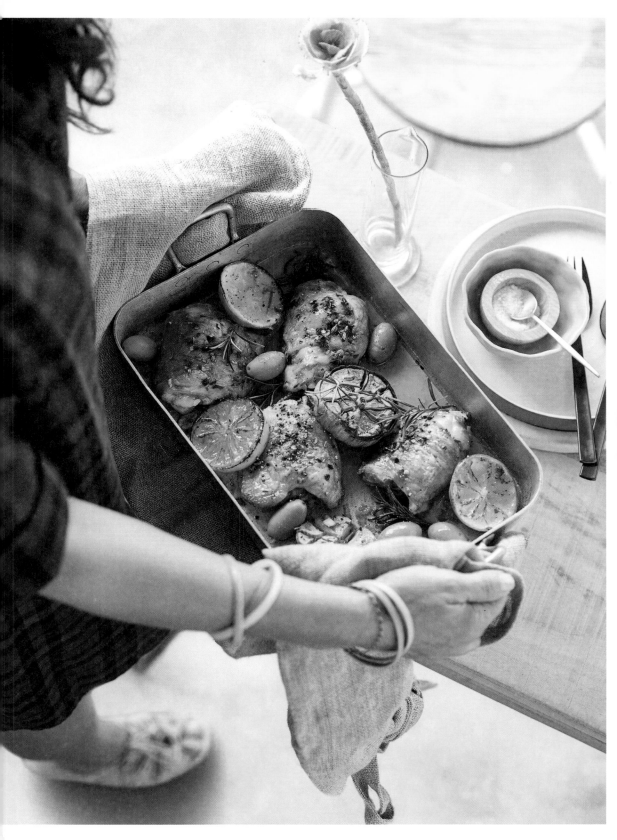

DR PEDRE'S CUBAN 'PICADILLO'

● GF   ● WF   ○ DF   ● SF

SERVES 2–3

This is a classic Cuban dish that Dr Pedre, who wrote the Foreword to this book, grew up with, watching his grandmother make it in the kitchen. He has reinvented it to be easy to digest, but still made with love. Rich in heart-healthy omega-3 fatty acids and coconut oil, this aromatic dish will fill your house with wonderful aromas and enrich your tastebuds with a virtual trip to the jewel of the Caribbean.

Steamed butternut pumpkin (squash) or baked sweet potato makes a lovely accompaniment, especially on a cold winter's night.

2 tablespoons extra virgin coconut oil
3 tablespoons dried herbes de Provence (thyme, rosemary, oregano and marjoram)
700 g (1 lb 9 oz) grass-fed minced (ground) beef, or free-range minced (ground) turkey
juice of 1 lemon
2 teaspoons garlic powder
1 tablespoon fresh thyme leaves
2 teaspoons ground turmeric
pinch of Himalayan or Celtic sea salt
85 g (3 oz/$\frac{1}{2}$ cup) pimento-stuffed olives
60 ml (2 fl oz/$\frac{1}{4}$ cup) apple cider vinegar
chopped parsley, to garnish

Melt the coconut oil in a large heavy-based saucepan over medium heat. Add the dried herbs and cook for 1 minute, or until aromatic.

Add the beef, breaking up the lumps with a wooden spoon, and cook until browned. Sprinkle with the lemon juice and garlic powder and stir well. Reduce the heat, cover and simmer for 5 minutes.

Sprinkle with the thyme, turmeric, salt and a good grind of black pepper. Stir well, breaking the beef up a bit more, if necessary. Add the olives and simmer for a further 5 minutes, stirring occasionally.

Stir in the vinegar, then reduce the heat to very low. Cover and cook for another 10–15 minutes, stirring now and then.

Serve sprinkled with chopped parsley, with your choice of accompaniment.

CHICKEN CROCKPOT WITH 25 GARLIC CLOVES

● GF ● WF ○ DF ● SF

SERVES 4

Garlic is a gloriously medicinal bulb to load up on for overall health. It's known to fight off infections, lower blood pressure, help remove lead from the body, and protect the heart against calcification and slow hardening of the arteries. Garlic is high in manganese, vitamin B6, vitamin C and selenium, and is also wonderful for gut health, killing pathogenic bacteria and feeding good bacteria. Believe me, 25 garlic cloves is never too much!

4 chicken thighs, on the bone, skin removed, about 900 g (2 lb) in total
1 tablespoon extra virgin olive oil
25 garlic cloves, peeled
2 small brown onions, roughly chopped
1 large eggplant (aubergine), cut into 3 cm (1¼ inch) chunks
1 large red capsicum (pepper), cut into 3 cm (1¼ inch) chunks
3 small dried shiitake mushrooms
2 tablespoons apple cider vinegar
2 tablespoons wheat-free tamari
500 ml (17 fl oz/2 cups) good-quality chicken broth or bone stock,
     such as the Gut-Healing Turmeric Chicken Broth on page 192

Place the chicken thighs in a slow cooker or crockpot. Drizzle with the olive oil and add all the remaining ingredients.

Put the lid on and cook for 6 hours at a low setting, or 3 hours on a high setting, until the chicken is very tender.

Cauliflower rice makes a lovely accompaniment.

 NOTE: *You can also bake the chicken in a covered casserole dish in a preheated 160°C (315°F) oven for 1½–2 hours.*

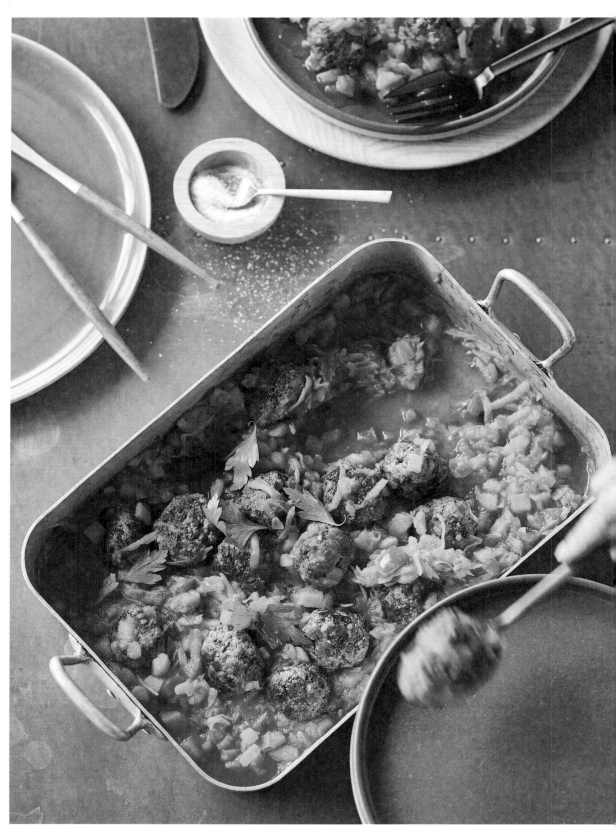

LOW-FODMAP MEATBALL STEW

● GF ● WF ○ DF ● SF

SERVES 4, OR UP TO 6 WITH A SIDE OF ZOODLES

Inspired by the flavours of Italy, here's a FODMAP-friendly meal the whole family will enjoy.

1 teaspoon garlic-infused extra virgin olive oil
4 spring onions (scallions), green tips only, roughly chopped
1 small sweet potato, peeled and cut into 2 cm (³/₄ inch) chunks
2 carrots, grated
1 red capsicum (pepper), chopped
500 g (1 lb 2 oz) very ripe roma (plum) tomatoes, chopped, reserving the juices
4 tablespoons tomato paste (concentrated purée)
125 ml (4 fl oz/¹/₂ cup) low-FODMAP stock

2 tablespoons lemon juice
2 tablespoons apple cider vinegar
roughly chopped parsley, to garnish

ITALIAN MEATBALLS

500 g (1 lb 2 oz) lean minced (ground) beef
1 tablespoon garlic-infused extra virgin olive oil
1 teaspoon ground oregano
1 bunch of flat-leaf (Italian) parsley, about 100 g (3¹/₂ oz), roughly chopped

Place all the meatball ingredients in a bowl and mix with your hands until well combined. Form into balls, about 4 cm (1¹/₂ inches) in diameter. Set aside.

Heat the olive oil in a heavy-based saucepan over medium heat. Add the meatballs and cook for about 8–10 minutes, turning now and then, until golden all over. Transfer the meatballs to a plate and set aside.

In the same pan, sauté the spring onion over medium heat for 2–3 minutes. Add the sweet potato, carrot, capsicum and tomatoes, including the tomato juices. Stir in the tomato paste, stock, lemon juice and vinegar.

Bring to the boil, then reduce the heat to low and simmer for 30 minutes, adding a little more stock or filtered water if necessary.

Add the browned meatballs and cook for a further 8–10 minutes, or until heated through, taking care not to overcook them, as you don't want them to become dry.

Season to taste with sea salt and freshly ground black pepper. Serve sprinkled with chopped parsley, with your choice of accompaniment.

HEARTY LAMB SHANKS WITH ROOT VEGIES & GREMOLATA

● GF ● WF ○ DF ● SF

SERVES 4

Here's a winter comfort stew that's full of flavour, and sure to salve and sustain a tender tummy.

2 tablespoons extra virgin olive oil
4 lamb shanks, about 1.25 kg
  (2 lb 12 oz) in total
2 carrots, roughly chopped
4 celery stalks, roughly chopped
4 garlic cloves, roughly chopped
750 ml (26 fl oz/3 cups) bone broth
  (see pages 192–198) or good-
  quality stock
4 thyme sprigs
1 small celeriac, peeled and diced

1 sweet potato, peeled and diced
2 parsnips, peeled and roughly
  chopped

GREMOLATA
1/2 cup roughly chopped flat-leaf
  (Italian) parsley
2 teaspoons grated lemon zest
1/4 garlic clove, crushed or
  finely grated

Heat half the olive oil in a large heavy-based saucepan over medium–high heat.

Season the shanks with sea salt and freshly ground black pepper. Working in batches, cook for 4–6 minutes, turning occasionally, until browned all over. Remove from the pan and set aside.

Add the remaining oil to the pan and sauté the carrot, celery and garlic for 3–4 minutes, or until softened.

Stir in the broth, then return the shanks to the pan. Add the thyme sprigs, celeriac, sweet potato and parsnip and bring to the boil.

Reduce the heat to low, then cover and simmer for 2–2 1/2 hours, or until the lamb is tender and falling off the bone, turning the shanks halfway through. If needed, stir in a little filtered water during cooking.

Remove the shanks from the pan. Remove the meat from the bones, break into bite-sized pieces and return them to the sauce. (Or leave the meat on the bone, if you prefer.)

Combine all the gremolata ingredients in a small bowl and serve sprinkled over the stew.

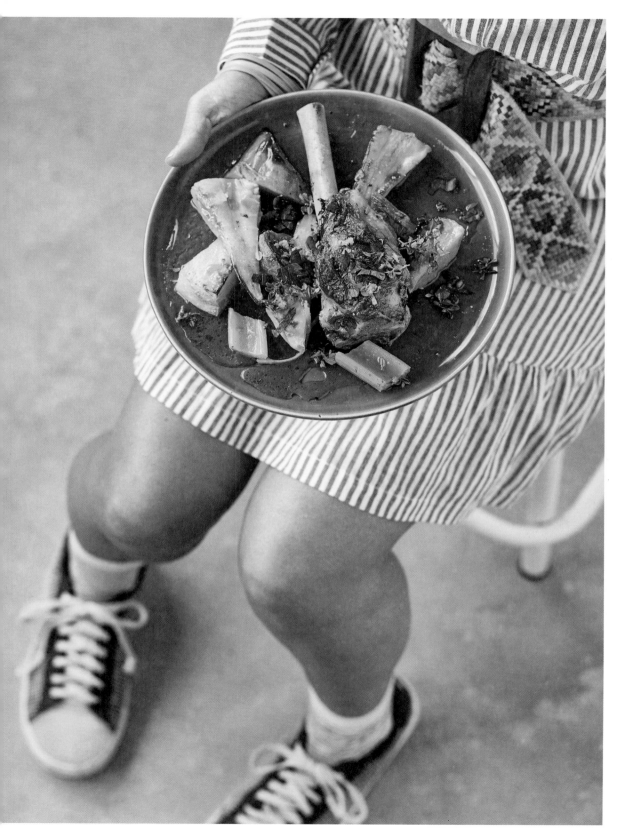

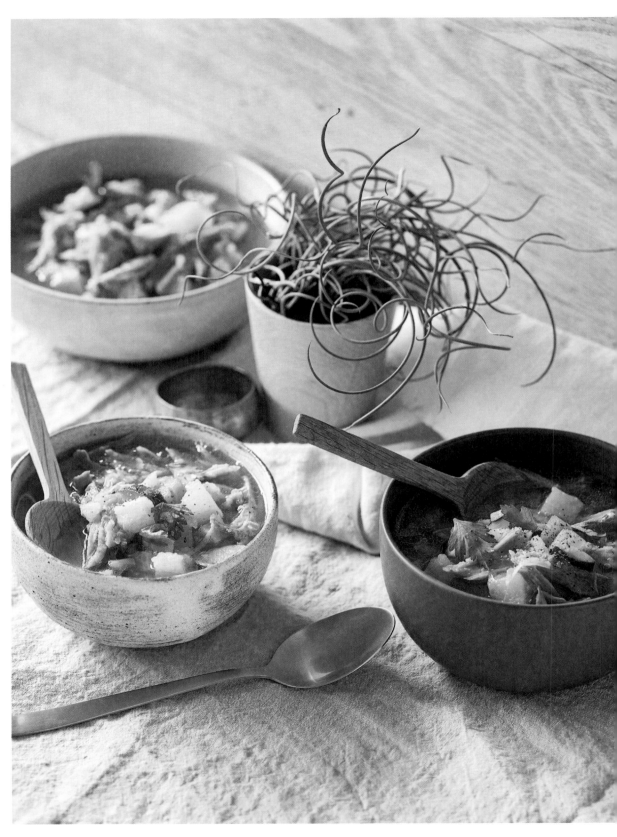

LOW-FODMAP SLOW-COOKED HAM HOCK SOUP

● GF ● WF ○ DF ● SF

SERVES 6

A hearty and harmonious FODMAP-friendly bowl of goodness awaits you, ready to turn those tummy troubles around.

1 tablespoon garlic-infused extra virgin olive oil
1 large turnip, peeled and diced
2 parsnips, peeled and diced
2 carrots, diced
4 celery stalks, sliced (optional; omit if not tolerated)
2 zucchini (courgettes), diced
1 small sweet potato, peeled and cut into 2 cm ($^3/_4$ inch) chunks
1 kg (2 lb 4 oz) organic, nitrate-free ham hock, skin scored to release the flavours
2 litres (68 fl oz/8 cups) low-FODMAP chicken stock
1 bay leaf
1 handful of parsley, roughly torn

Heat the olive oil in a large heavy-based saucepan over medium–low heat. Add the vegetables, season with sea salt and freshly ground black pepper and cook, stirring regularly, for 15 minutes.

Add the ham hock and pour in the stock. Add the bay leaf and bring to the boil, then reduce the heat to low. Simmer for 1½–2 hours to allow the flavours to develop, skimming off any foam that rises to the surface, and topping up with extra stock or filtered water if needed.

Leave to cool slightly, then carefully remove the hock from the pan and place on a chopping board. Pull the meat from the bone, shred the meat and add it to the soup. Remove the bay leaf and season to taste.

Serve warm, topped with the parsley.

SUPERCHARGED TIP

This soup can be portioned into airtight containers and frozen for deliciously convenient meals.

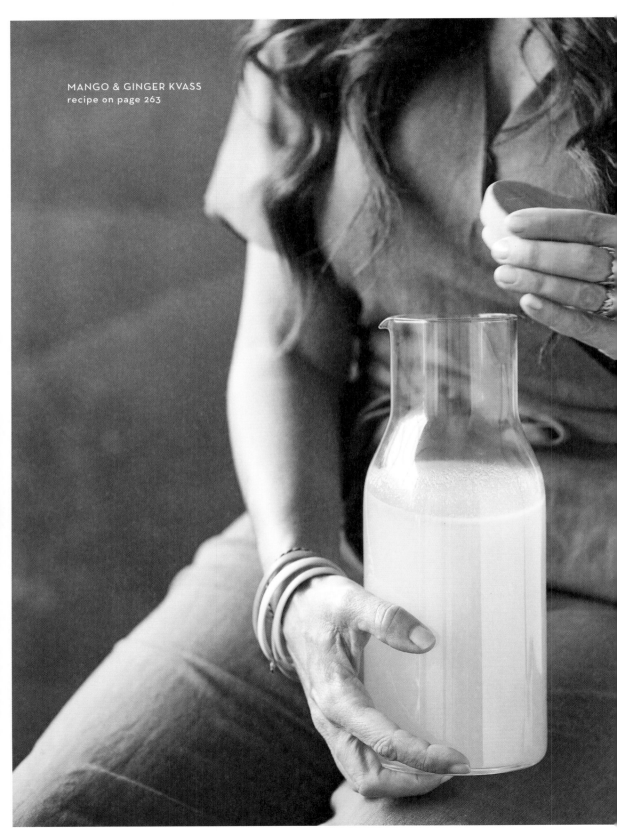

MANGO & GINGER KVASS
recipe on page 263

CULTURE CLUB

Cultivate your inner ecosystem with friendly ferments designed to enhance digestion and boost immunity. Kraut, kvass and kefir lovers, your kitchen time starts now.

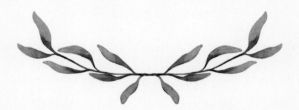

COCONUT MILK KEFIR

● GF ● WF ○ DF ● SF ● VEG

MAKES ABOUT 375 ML (13 FL OZ/1½ CUPS)

This delicious drink is beneficial for your tummy and tastes like liquid yoghurt. Kefir contains beneficial yeast and friendly probiotic bacteria, maintaining the friendly bacterial in the gut.

You can buy kefir grains online, and from health food shops.

**1 tablespoon milk kefir grains, or 2 probiotic capsules,
or 1 teaspoon probiotic powder
375 ml (13 fl oz/1½ cups) Coconut Milk (page 137),
at room temperature
liquid stevia or stevia powder, to taste (optional)**

You'll need a sterilised 500 ml (17 fl oz/2 cup) mason jar with lid, a wooden spoon, some muslin (cheesecloth), an elastic band and a nylon strainer; avoid using metal implements.

Pour the coconut milk into the mason jar, add the kefir grains and give the mixture a quick stir with a wooden spoon.

Cover the jar with muslin and secure with an elastic band.

Leave to sit in a cool, dry, dark place for about 24 hours to ferment.

Your kefir will be ready when it tastes effervescent and sour, and there is no remaining sweetness.

Strain the kefir through a nylon strainer (you might have to jiggle it a bit). Add stevia to taste, if you like.

Pour into a sterilised glass bottle and transfer to the fridge to thicken slightly, where it will keep for up to 2 weeks.

Enjoy it with breakfast bowls, in smoothies, or with Fermented Berries (see page 268).

SUPERCHARGED TIP

You can use the leftover kefir grains again — just place them in a clean mason jar and repeat the process by adding more coconut milk.

MANGO & GINGER KVASS

● GF ● WF ● DF

MAKES ABOUT 500 ML (17 FL OZ/2 CUPS)

A refreshingly nourishing blend of probiotic and enzyme-rich sweetness and tartness, kvass is a fantastic alternative to soft drinks. You can vary the flavour using different fruits, such as apples, berries and pineapples. Bottoms up!

The culture starter is optional if using tap water, and can be purchased online or from a health food store.

2 ripe mangoes, peeled and chopped
2.5 cm (1 inch) knob of fresh ginger, grated
1 tablespoon raw honey
culture starter (optional, if using tap water; check the packet instructions
    for the recommended quantity to use)
filtered water, to almost fill the jar

Place the mango and ginger in a sterilised 1 litre (35 fl oz/4 cup) mason jar and drizzle in the honey. Add the starter culture, if using.

Pour enough filtered water into the jar to cover the mixture, but leaving about 2.5 cm (1 inch) of breathing space at the top of the jar, to allow the pressure to build.

Cover the jar with plastic wrap, then screw the lid on tightly. Leave to sit on the counter for 2 days, shaking the jar periodically.

After 24–48 hours, you should notice some bubbles. After 24 hours, you can 'burp' your brew by opening the lid carefully and then retightening it. This will allow carbon dioxide to be released, so you don't have an explosion!

On day two, check your fruit to ensure it is bubbling. It should taste slightly tangy.

Strain the fruit, pour the kvass into a sterilised glass bottle and store in the fridge. It will keep for 3–4 days.

SUPERCHARGED TIP

Most fruits can be left to ferment for up to 7 days, but soft fruits such as banana, mango and papaya can be ready in 2 days. It's best not to over-ferment them, as they can become very sour.

CULTURED VEGETABLES

● GF   ● WF   ● DF   ● SF   ● VEG

MAKES 2 X 1 LITRE (35 FL OZ/4 CUP) MASON JARS

Once you get to learn the process, fermenting can be lots of fun. Start by choosing vegetables you're familiar with, so it doesn't feel intimidating.

Fermented vegetables can be served as a side dish — just start with a small amount, such as a teaspoonful, and work your way up.

4 carrots, peeled and diced
4 celery stalks, chopped
500 g (1 lb 2 oz/4 cups) cauliflower florets
1 red or yellow capsicum (pepper), chopped or sliced
3 tablespoons grated fresh ginger
2 garlic cloves, chopped
90 g (3¼ oz/⅔ cup) Celtic sea salt
filtered water, to cover

Combine the vegetables, ginger and garlic in a sturdy bowl. Pound them with a pestle or rolling pin until slightly smashed and softened.

Add the salt and toss well. Press the mixture into two sterilised 1 litre (35 fl oz) mason jars, leaving about 2.5 cm (1 inch) of breathing space at the top of each jar, to allow for expansion.

Pour in enough water to just cover the vegetables, adding more salt if needed to submerge them — the mixture needs to be very salty.

Cover the jars with plastic wrap, then screw the lids on tightly. Leave to ferment in a warm place for 3–5 days.

Do a taste test until you're pleased with the flavour, removing any mould that may form on the surface. The vegetables should taste tangy.

Store in the fridge and use within 1 week.

 NOTE: *To sterilise jars and lids, you can run them through a dishwasher, or wash them in clean soapy water, rinse well and dry them in a low oven.*

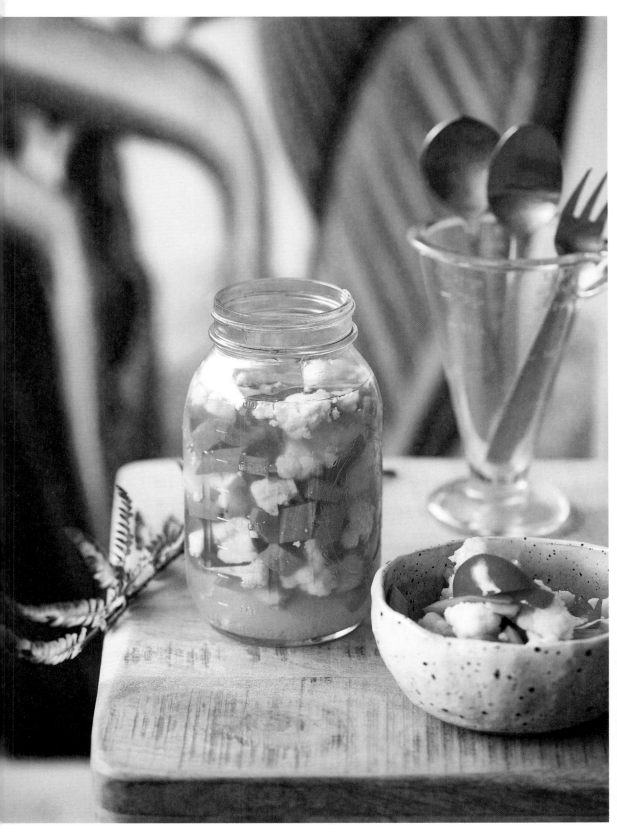

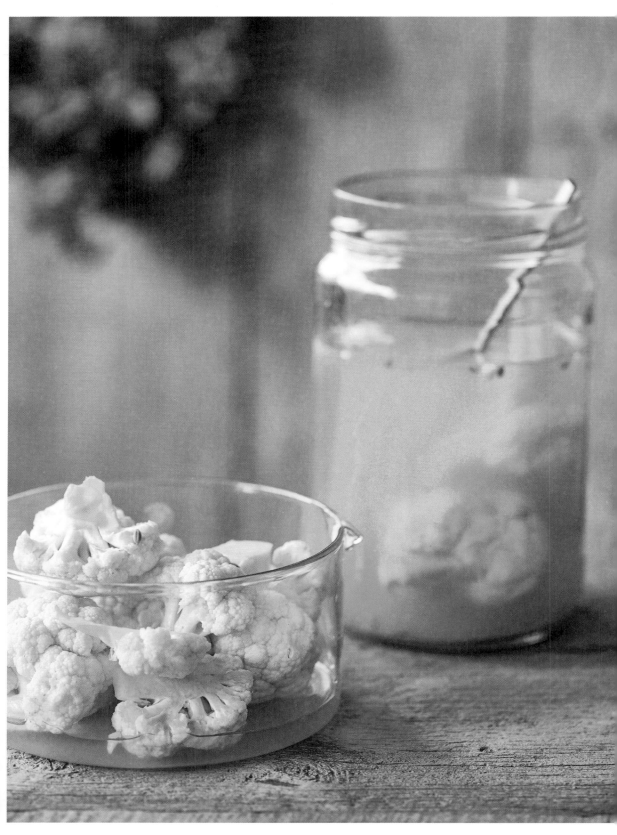

TURMERIC & FENNEL CAULIFLOWER

● GF ● WF ○ DF ● SF ● VEG

MAKES 1 X 1 LITRE (35 FL OZ/4 CUP) MASON JAR

Take cauliflower to new heights in this colourful Indian-spiced ferment.

1 head of cauliflower, cut into florets
½ teaspoon ground turmeric
½ teaspoon fennel seeds
2 tablespoons Celtic sea salt
500 ml (17 fl oz/2 cups) filtered water

Place the cauliflower, turmeric and fennel seeds in a bowl. Toss to mix the spices through the cauliflower.

Transfer the mixture to a sterilised 1 litre (35 fl oz/4 cup) mason jar, pressing down to remove any large air gaps, and leaving about 2.5 cm (1 inch) of headroom at the top.

Dissolve the salt in the filtered water, then pour it over the cauliflower, ensuring it is fully submerged, and leaving about 2.5 cm (1 inch) of breathing room at the top of the jar, to allow for expansion.

Cover the jar with plastic wrap, then screw the lid on tightly.

Keep in a warm place for 3–4 days, then open and taste test until you're satisfied with the result; the vegetables should taste tangy.

Store in the fridge and use within 3–5 days.

FERMENTED BERRIES

● GF ● WF ● DF

MAKES 1 X 500 ML (17 FL OZ/2 CUP) MASON JAR

A versatile gut-loving ingredient, fermented fruits and berries are soft, puffy and slightly sweet, and can be mashed or puréed into sauces to drizzle over baked custard, nicecream (pages 282–286), breakfast oats and yoghurt. You'll also love them in popsicles (pages 288–289), or on top of pancakes and crepes.

400 g (14 oz/2 cups) fresh mixed berries
2–3 tablespoons filtered water
2 tablespoons raw honey
1/2 teaspoon starter culture (sold online and at health food stores. Follow packet instructions for quantity needed as they vary.)
1/4 teaspoon Celtic sea salt

Place the berries in a sterilised 500 ml (17 fl oz/2 cup) mason jar, packing them tightly with a wooden spoon to remove any air gaps, and leaving about 2.5 cm (1 inch) of headroom at the top.

In a small sterilised jug, mix together the remaining ingredients until the salt has dissolved.

Pour the liquid over the berries, ensuring they are submerged, and leaving about 2.5 cm (1 inch) of breathing room at the top of the jar, to allow for expansion.

Cover the jar with plastic wrap, then screw the lid on tightly.

Store at room temperature for 1–2 days, or until bubbles start to form.

Transfer to the fridge, where the berries will keep for up to 4 weeks.

 NOTE: *Covering the top of the jar with plastic wrap before screwing the lid on stops the metal of the lid coming in contact with the fermenting liquid.*

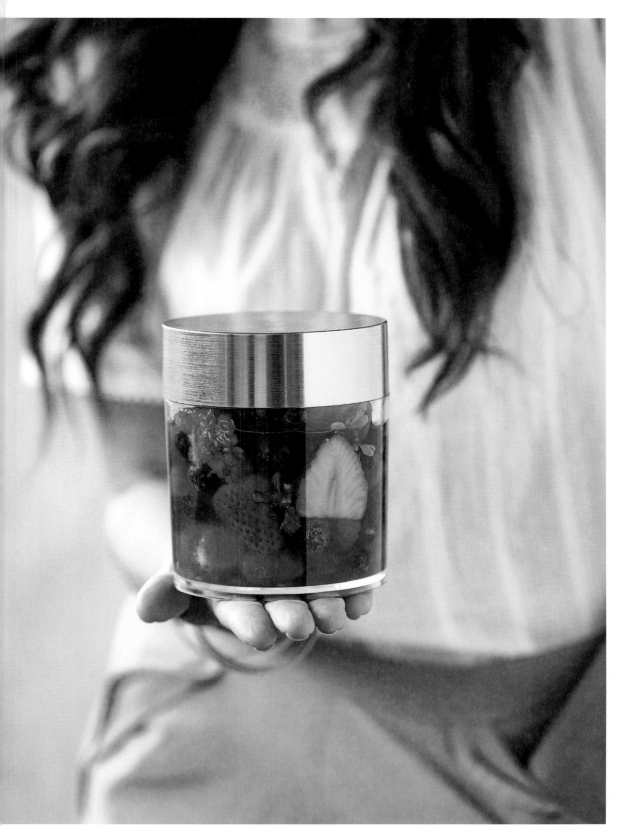

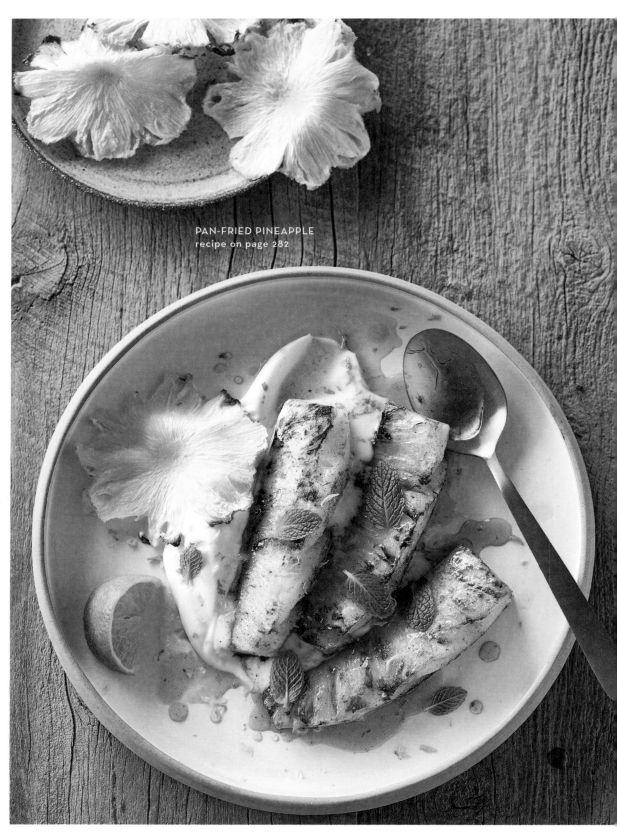

PAN-FRIED PINEAPPLE
recipe on page 282

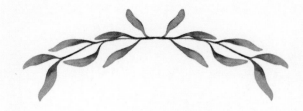

DESSERTS WITH BENEFITS

The following pages are proof that gut-friendly indulgences come with a multitude of benefits. These are treats you can enjoy without twisting your tummy up in knots. You'll even find cauliflower transformed into a sweet and creamy dessert, with a bonus raspberry ripple swirled through.

RASPBERRY PEPPERMINT BARK

● GF ● WF ○ DF ● VEG

SERVES 4

Move over candy canes, my no-bake peppermint raspberry bark is the newest treat to take the holidays by storm.

3 tablespoons organic coconut butter
1 tablespoon extra virgin coconut oil
400 ml (14 fl oz) tin coconut cream
pinch of Celtic sea salt
1 teaspoon peppermint oil
1 teaspoon alcohol-free vanilla extract
40 g (1½ oz/⅓ cup) fresh or frozen raspberries
2 tablespoons flaked coconut (optional)

Melt the coconut butter and coconut oil in a heatproof bowl, over a saucepan of boiling water. Add the coconut cream, salt, peppermint oil and vanilla, stirring to combine.

Pour onto a tray lined with baking paper, then evenly scatter the raspberries over, and the shredded coconut, if using.

Freeze for 1 hour, or until solid. Break into shards, or chop into squares. Store in an airtight container in the freezer, where it will keep for up to 2 weeks.

SUPERCHARGED TIP

To make **Turmeric Tummy Bark**, place 80 ml (2½ oz/⅓ cup) extra virgin coconut oil in a high-speed blender. Add 3 tablespoons organic coconut butter, 1 teaspoon ground turmeric, a pinch of freshly ground black pepper, a pinch of vanilla powder, 1 tablespoon rice malt syrup (or liquid stevia, to taste), and as an optional extra, 1 tablespoon pure food-grade diatomaceous earth (see page 43), such as my Love Your Gut Powder. Whiz until smooth. Stir in 45 g (1½ oz/⅓ cup) slivered almonds. Spread the mixture over a tray lined with baking paper. Freeze for 1 hour, or until set. Enjoy straight from freezer. To serve, break into handy pieces and bite-sized snacks.

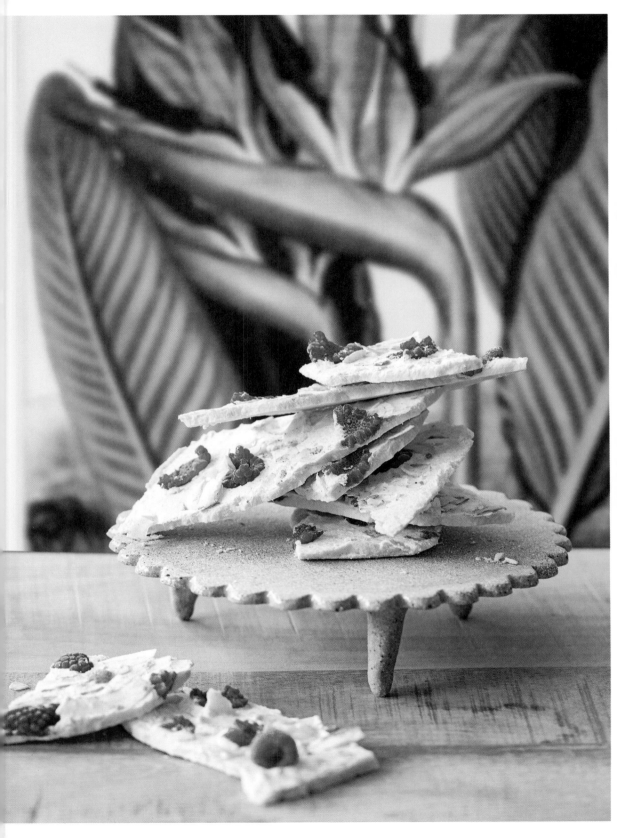

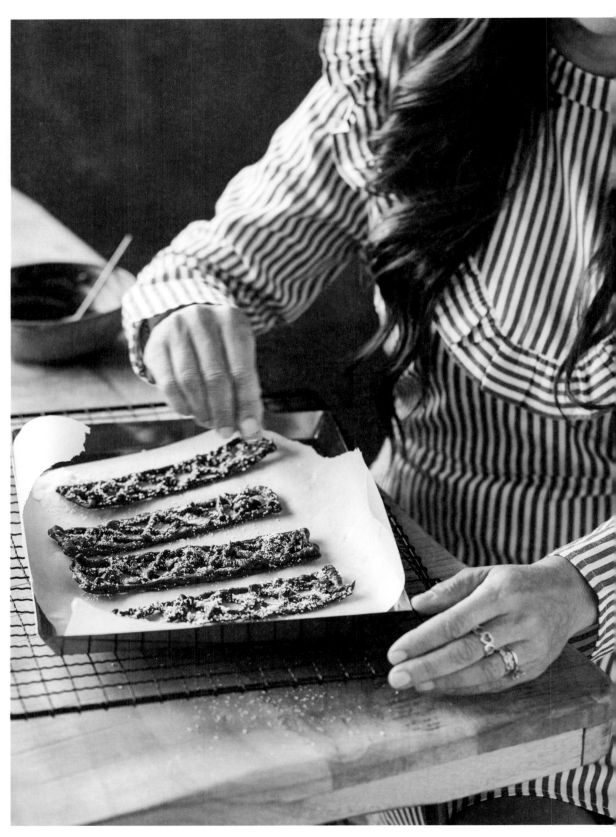

CHOCOLATE CURLS

● GF ● WF ● DF ● VEG (IF NOT USING HONEY)

SERVES 4

This gut-friendly sweet treat offers so much flavour and chocolatey fun!
It's a great one to make and enjoy with kids.

240 g (8½ oz/1 cup) cacao butter
30 g (1 oz/¼ cup) raw cacao powder, sifted
1 teaspoon vanilla powder
1 heaped teaspoon maca powder
2 tablespoons rice malt syrup or raw honey,
    or 1 teaspoon liquid stevia
25 g (1 oz/¼ cup) desiccated coconut

Line a baking tray with baking paper.

Melt the cacao butter in a heatproof bowl, over a saucepan of boiling water,
stirring constantly.

Stir in the cacao powder, vanilla powder, maca powder and rice malt syrup or
raw honey (or the stevia) until combined. Set aside until thick enough to pipe.

Pour the mixture into a piping (icing) bag and pipe it onto the baking paper,
in a squiggly pattern, forming fingers about 15 cm (6 inches) long, and leaving
space in between. (Alternatively, use a skewer to drag the mixture across the
paper to create a pattern.)

Top with the coconut and place in the fridge for about 1 hour to harden.

It will keep in an airtight container in the fridge for 2–3 weeks.

APPLE CIDER GUMMY BEARS

● GF ● WF ● DF

MAKES ABOUT 12

Finally, a yummy gummy that's good for your tummy. Bring it on.

250 ml (9 fl oz/1 cup) apple juice (no added sugar)
60 ml (2 fl oz/¼ cup) apple cider vinegar
3 tablespoons powdered gelatine

In a small saucepan, warm the apple juice and vinegar over medium heat.
    When it starts to bubble, remove from the heat.
    Sprinkle the gelatine on top and whisk briskly until dissolved. Strain.
    Pour into teddy bear moulds, or other moulds of your choice, or into
a small lined baking tin. Refrigerate for 1–2 hours, or until set.
    Turn out of the moulds, or cut into small squares to serve. The gummies
will keep in an airtight container in the fridge or freezer for 1–2 weeks.

SUPERCHARGED TIP

*To make **Aloe Vera Gummies**, replace the vinegar with aloe vera juice.*
*For **Vegetarian Gummies**, simply heat up 350 ml (12 fl oz) aloe vera juice in*
a saucepan, add ½ teaspoon agar-agar flakes or powder and stir to dissolve.
Continue stirring for a couple of minutes. When the mixture starts to boil,
remove from the heat, add some liquid stevia, vanilla extract, chopped
mint or whatever spice you like — even berries would be nice! Pour into
an ice-cube tray. Top with shredded coconut if you like, then refrigerate
for about 1 hour, or until set.

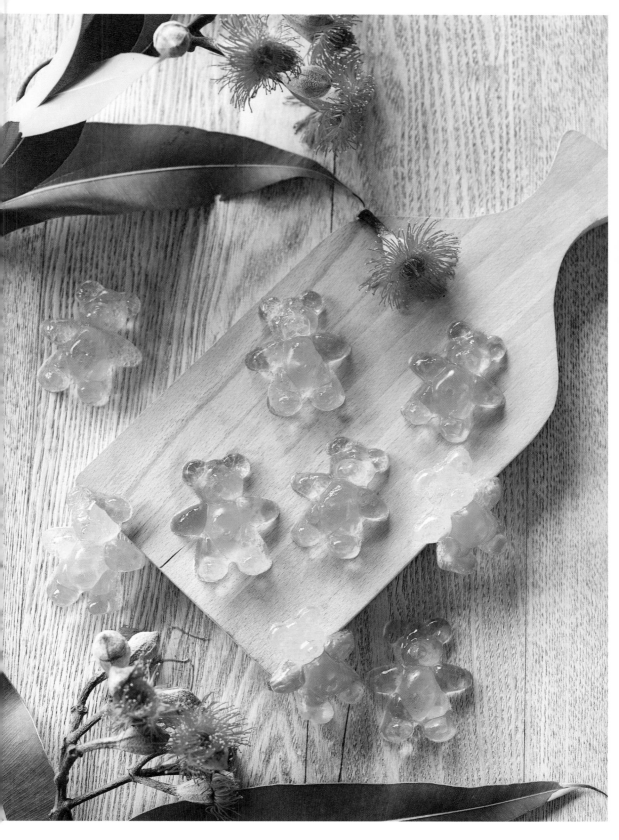

LICORICE & RASPBERRY JELLY

● GF ● WF ○ DF

SERVES 2–3

This fabulous jelly is ultra-healing for the gut lining. It's filled with gelatine, a gut-supporting superstar that provides essential amino acids to heal and seal the gut lining, reduce inflammation and improve digestion — assisted by liquorice root, a herb often taken to soothe digestive complaints such as stomach ulcers, heartburn, colic and leaky gut.

Even better, this jelly is also free of added sugar, relying on the natural sweetness of vitamin C-rich raspberries and stevia.

A brilliant way to boost gut health in the form of a seemingly naughty treat that the kids will adore!

500 ml (17 fl oz/2 cups) filtered water
90 g (3½ oz/¾ cup) frozen raspberries
1 liquorice tea bag (or other herbal tea bag of your choice)
2 tablespoons lemon juice
small pinch of Celtic sea salt
½ teaspoon liquid stevia, or to taste
80 ml (2½ fl oz/⅓ cup) warm filtered water
4 teaspoons powdered gelatine
40 g (1½ oz/⅓ cup) fresh raspberries, cut in half

Pour the filtered water into a small saucepan.
Add the frozen raspberries and tea bag and bring to a gentle simmer.
Remove from the heat and allow the tea to steep for a few minutes.

Strain into a jug, stir in the lemon juice and salt, and add stevia to taste.

Pour the warm filtered water into a bowl and sprinkle the gelatine on top. Stir for about 1 minute, until the gelatine has dissolved. Strain into the steeped tea mixture and stir until combined.

Pour into a jelly mould or container of choice, and add the fresh raspberries. Chill in the refrigerator for about 3 hours, or until set.

The jelly will keep in the fridge for 3–5 days.

TURMERIC FUDGE

● GF ● WF ○ DF ● VEG

MAKES 10–12 SLICES

A super-fun, one-bowl masterpiece full of golden, fudgy goodness!

140 g (5 oz/½ cup) tahini
60 ml (2 fl oz/¼ cup) rice malt syrup
60 ml (2 fl oz/¼ cup) melted extra virgin coconut oil
2 tablespoons food-grade diatomaceous earth (see page 43),
   such as my Love Your Gut Powder (optional)
2 teaspoons ground turmeric
1 teaspoon ground ginger

Line a small 15 cm (6 inch) square baking dish with baking paper.
   Combine all the ingredients in a bowl, mixing well, then pour into the
baking dish. Set in the fridge for about 1 hour.
   Cut into slices to serve.
   The fudge will keep in an airtight container in the fridge for up to 1 week.

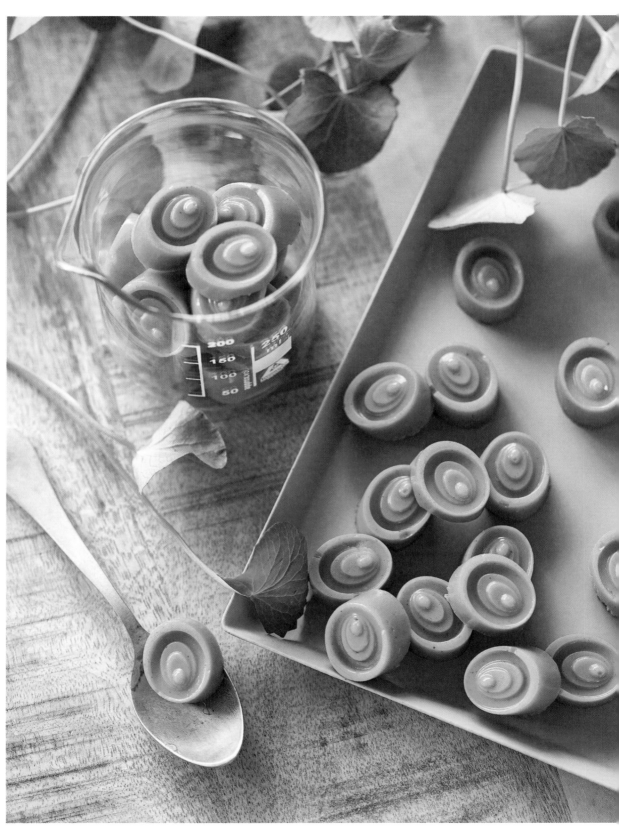

TURMERIC TUMMY GUMMIES

● GF ● WF ● DF

MAKES 20–30

Loaded with turmeric and its botanical cousin ginger, these delicious gummy treats can help settle your digestive system and reduce inflammation in the body. As well as being a wonderful immunity booster and de-bloater, ginger helps to reduce nausea and is also an appetite suppressant, while turmeric is a powerful antioxidant that can also aid in weight maintenance. Think of this dazzling duo as an inflammation-squashing combination that can be sprinkled into many of your favourite meals, and made into soothing hot drinks. Black pepper is also included in these gorgeous gummies as it helps to improve the absorption of curcumin, the active component of turmeric, by your body.

60 ml (2 fl oz/¼ cup) warm filtered water
2 tablespoons powdered gelatine
250 ml (9 fl oz/1 cup) Coconut Milk (page 137)
1 tablespoon ground turmeric
1 teaspoon ground ginger
good pinch of freshly ground black pepper
1 teaspoon food-grade diatomaceous earth (see page 43),
    such as my Love Your Gut Powder (optional), or see Note
3 tablespoons rice malt syrup, or raw honey

Pour the filtered water into a large bowl and sprinkle the gelatine over. Set aside until it starts to 'bloom'.

Place the remaining ingredients in a saucepan and warm over low heat for about 5 minutes. Whisk until well combined. Slowly whisk the coconut milk mixture into the gelatine mixture. Continue whisking to remove any lumps.

Strain, then pour into moulds, or a lined baking tin or dish.

Chill in the refrigerator for 3 hours, or until firm enough to turn out out of the moulds, or to slice into cubes. The gummies will keep in an airtight container in the fridge for up to 1 week.

 NOTE: *You can also use 1 tablespoon of my Golden Gut Blend for this recipe (see Appendix). It's an organic blend of diatomaceous earth, turmeric, ginger, cinnamon and black pepper. If using in these gummies, omit the Love Your Gut Powder here as well as the ginger, turmeric and pepper – these ingredients are all contained in the blend. It's also amazing in smoothies, lattes and nicecreams – even curries or casseroles. So versatile!*

PAN-FRIED PINEAPPLE

● GF ● WF ○ DF ● VEG

SERVES 2–3

A simply luscious blend of caramelised sweetness and coconut yoghurt.

2 tablespoons extra virgin coconut oil
6 pineapple wedges, skin removed
zest and juice of 1 lime
250 g (9 oz/1 cup) coconut yoghurt
mint leaves, to garnish

Melt the coconut oil in a heavy-based frying pan over medium heat.

Add the pineapple, drizzle with the lime juice and cook for 4–5 minutes on each side, or until golden brown.

Serve warm, with coconut yoghurt, garnished with the mint and lime zest.

SALTED CARAMEL NICECREAM

● GF ● WF ○ DF ● VEG

SERVES 1–2

Ice-cream lovers, I have you covered. My salted caramel nicecream is here!

2 frozen bananas, peeled and
   roughly chopped
2 teaspoons hulled tahini
1 tablespoon smooth nut butter
   (cashew is good)

$\frac{1}{4}$ teaspoon ground cinnamon,
   plus extra to serve
$\frac{1}{2}$ teaspoon vanilla powder
$\frac{1}{8}$ teaspoon Celtic sea salt
1 teaspoon maca powder (optional)

Place the banana in a high-speed blender. Add the tahini, nut butter, cinnamon, vanilla powder, salt and maca, if using. Whiz until smooth and creamy.

Serve immediately, with an extra sprinkling of cinnamon.

For a firmer nicecream, freeze for 4 hours, or until set, then scoop into bowls or cones; if it becomes too hard to scoop, place in the fridge to soften.

BERRY RIPPLE CAULIFLOWER NICECREAM

● GF ● WF ● DF ● VEG

SERVES 2–3

Yes, it's true: cauliflower can be transformed into a sweet, creamy dessert! Combined with easily digestible bananas and creamy soaked cashews, this frozen delight is a sneaky way to increase your kids' vegie count in a way they'd never suspect. This nicecream is gorgeous made into a sundae topped with all kinds of healthy sprinkles, ranging from chia seeds to chopped macadamia nuts, cacao nibs and my favourite, Fermented Berries (page 268).

For a chocolate version, add 1$\frac{1}{2}$ tablespoons raw cacao powder. To make a berry ripple version, add 2 tablespoons of the Berry Coulis (see below) and swirl it through.

$\frac{1}{2}$ head of cauliflower, cut into small florets
2 bananas, peeled and roughly chopped, plus extra sliced banana to serve
165 g (5$\frac{3}{4}$ oz/1 cup) natural cashews, soaked in filtered water for 3–4 hours, then strained
400 ml (14 fl oz) tin coconut milk, chilled
1 teaspoon vanilla powder

$\frac{1}{8}$ teaspoon Celtic sea salt
6–8 drops of liquid stevia, or to taste

BERRY COULIS

200 g (7 oz/1$\frac{1}{2}$ cups) frozen berries, thawed
8 drops of liquid stevia
1 teaspoon apple cider vinegar (optional)

Place the cauliflower in a saucepan and cover with water. Bring to the boil and cook for about 10–15 minutes, or until very tender. Drain, leave to cool, then place in a high-speed blender with the banana, cashews, coconut milk, vanilla and salt. Whiz until smooth, then sweeten to taste with stevia.

Transfer to a container and place in the freezer to set for 1–2 hours; it will keep for up to 1 week.

This nicecream does set very hard, so remove it from the freezer for at least 15 minutes before serving, to allow it to soften.

To make the berry coulis, warm the berries and stevia in a saucepan over medium heat. Remove from the heat, add the vinegar if desired, then purée into a thick sauce using a hand-held stick blender. If you can, strain through a fine-meshed sieve to remove the seeds.

Serve the nicecream with the berry coulis and extra sliced banana.

MANGO NICECREAM

● GF   ● WF   ○ DF   ● VEG

SERVES 1–2

This enzymatic dessert is a delightful palate cleanser after a hearty meat dish, or as an afternoon pick-me-up on a hot summer's day.

Fresh mango is a fruit bursting with antioxidants, and over 20 different vitamins and minerals, and is a good source of fibre to keep you regular. Berries are rich in antioxidants and vitamin C for immune health, and contain tannins, which are thought to play a health-promoting role in the digestive tract by reducing inflammation.

½ large mango, diced and frozen (or use frozen mango chunks)
1 frozen banana, peeled and roughly chopped
125 ml (4 fl oz/½ cup) Coconut Milk (page 137)
125 g (4½ oz/½ cup) coconut yoghurt

½ teaspoon alcohol-free vanilla extract or vanilla powder
juice of 1 small lime
pinch of ground cinnamon
1 handful of blueberries, to serve (optional)
pinch of grated lime zest

Place the mango and banana in a high-speed blender. Add the coconut milk, coconut yoghurt, vanilla, lime juice and cinnamon. Whiz until smooth.

Serve immediately, topped with the blueberries, if using, and a sprinkling of lime zest.

For a firmer nicecream, freeze for 4 hours, or until set, then scoop into bowls or cones; if it becomes too hard to scoop, place in the fridge to soften.

SALTED CARAMEL NICECREAM
recipe on page 282

MANGO NICECREAM

GOLDEN NICECREAM

● GF ● WF ○ DF ● VEG

SERVES 4

Say goodbye to boring old vanilla ice cream and behold my golden take on a creamy dessert that'll have you breezing through spring and summer without a care in the world.

2 frozen bananas, peeled and roughly chopped
pinch of Celtic sea salt
⅛ teaspoon freshly ground black pepper
½ teaspoon ground cinnamon, plus extra to serve
½ teaspoon ground ginger
¼ teaspoon ground cardamom
2 teaspoons ground turmeric
1 teaspoon alcohol-free vanilla extract or vanilla powder
60 ml (2 fl oz/¼ cup) chilled Coconut Milk (page 137)
6 drops of liquid stevia, or 2 tablespoons rice malt syrup
fresh banana slices, to serve

Place the frozen banana in a high-speed blender. Add the salt and all the spices, the vanilla, coconut milk and your choice of sweetener.

Whiz until smooth. Serve immediately, topped with fresh banana and an extra sprinkling of cinnamon.

For a firmer nicecream, freeze for 4 hours, or until set, then scoop into bowls or cones; if it becomes too hard to scoop, place in the fridge to soften.

COCONUT & MANGO PANNA COTTA

● GF ● WF ● DF

SERVES 4

Deliciously decadent and refreshingly simple, this dairy-free dessert is bursting with flavour.

60 ml (2 fl oz/¼ cup) warm filtered water
1 teaspoon powdered gelatine
250 ml (9 fl oz/1 cup) Coconut Milk (page 137)
1 teaspoon vanilla powder
2 ripe mangoes, 1 puréed (see Note), 1 peeled and diced
torn mint leaves, to garnish

Pour the filtered water into a small bowl. Sprinkle the gelatine on top and mix well until completely dissolved.

In a separate bowl, mix together the coconut milk and vanilla powder. Strain the gelatine mixture into the bowl, then add the mango purée and mix well.

Spoon the mixture into four ramekins or short jars. Cover and chill in the fridge for 3–4 hours, until set.

Serve cold, topped with diced mango and torn mint leaves.

 NOTE: *To purée the mango, cut the cheeks off, scoop the flesh into a food processor and whiz until smooth.*

MATCHA POPSICLES

● GF   ○ WF   ○ DF   ● VEG

MAKES 6

All you need to make popsicles is a stick, a freezer, and a little imagination.

2 teaspoons matcha powder
400 ml (14 fl oz) tin coconut milk
80 ml (2½ fl oz/⅓ cup) rice malt syrup
1 teaspoon vanilla extract

Whisk all the ingredients together in a blender.
   Pour into popsicle (ice lolly) moulds and freeze for 4–6 hours,
inserting a popsicle stick in each when the mixture is almost set.
   These popsicles will keep in the freezer for up to 1 week.

COCONUT MOJITO POPSICLES

● GF   ○ WF   ○ DF   ◐ SF   ● VEG

MAKES 6–8

These no-fail popsicles are one of the best summer recipes I know of.
For the minimal amount of effort required to whip up a batch of these
darlings, it never ceases to amaze me how many times they've brought a
sense of delight to both adults and children on a sweltering summer's day.

2 tablespoons sliced mint leaves
grated zest and juice of 1 lime
6 drops of liquid stevia
500 ml (17 fl oz/2 cups) coconut water

Mix all the ingredients together in a jug.
   Pour into popsicle (ice lolly) moulds and freeze for 2–3 hours,
inserting a popsicle stick in each when the mixture is almost set.
   These popsicles will keep in the freezer for up to 1 week.

COCONUT POPSICLES

● GF ● WF ○ DF ● SF ● VEG

MAKES 6–8

In the searing heat of summer, you'll love these coconut popicles. They're refreshing, full of supercharged ingredients, and speedy to prepare.

2 x 400 ml (14 fl oz) tins organic coconut milk
seeds from 1 vanilla bean, or 1 teaspoon alcohol-free
    vanilla extract or vanilla powder
2 tablespoons food-grade diatomaceous earth (see page 43),
    such as my Love Your Gut Powder (optional)
10 drops of liquid stevia, or to taste

Put all the ingredients in a high-speed blender and whiz until smooth.
    Pour into popsicle (ice lolly) moulds and freeze for 3–4 hours, inserting a popsicle stick in each when the mixture is almost set.
    These popsicles are best eaten soon afterwards — if left overnight or too long in the freezer, the coconut milk sometimes splits.

SUPERCHARGED TIP

For **Choc-Coco Popsicles**, add 1 tablespoon raw cacao powder.

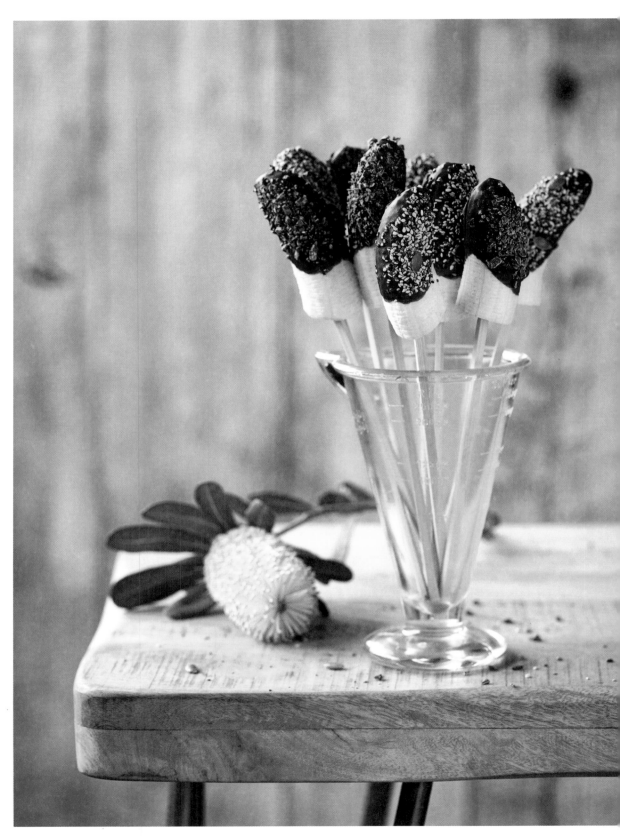

CHOCOLATE BANANAS ON STICKS

● GF ● WF ○ DF ● VEG

MAKES 8

The good bacteria in your gut love anti-inflammatory cacao and prebiotic-rich bananas — and so will your whole family! Serve these sticks of choc-coated deliciousness plain, or twirl them in your choice of extra toppings. They're perfect for whipping up during holidays.

4 bananas
40 g (1½ oz) cacao butter
3 tablespoons organic coconut butter
2 tablespoons extra virgin coconut oil
30 g (1 oz/¼ cup) raw cacao powder
1 teaspoon alcohol-free vanilla extract
10–12 drops of liquid stevia, or 1 teaspoon powdered
   stevia, or to taste

OPTIONAL TOPPINGS
toasted seeds and nuts (if tolerated)
shredded coconut flakes
cacao nibs
a drizzle of melted nut butter

Line a small tray with baking paper.
   Peel the bananas and cut in half across the middle. Place a popsicle stick or a thick bamboo skewer in each banana half and set aside.
   Melt the cacao butter, coconut butter and coconut oil in a heatproof bowl, over a saucepan of boiling water. Add the cacao powder, vanilla extract and stevia and whisk until smooth.
   Pour the chocolate sauce into a tall heatproof glass.
   Place your chosen toppings, if using, in a shallow bowl.
   One by one, dip the bananas in the chocolate sauce, ensuring they are well covered all the way around. You may need to dip them in the chocolate several times, freezing briefly between each dip, to give them a good coating.
   Dip the bananas in your toppings and place on the lined tray. Refrigerate for 30 minutes, or until the chocolate has hardened.
   Enjoy straight away, before they discolour, or freeze for up to 1 week.

APPENDIX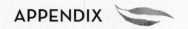

THE SUPERCHARGE YOUR GUT PROGRAM

I hope you've enjoyed the information and recipes in this book.
If you'd like to continue supercharging your gut, there are new recipes
appearing every week on my blog. The Supercharge Your Gut
maintenance program can also be continued online, with brand-new
recipes, weekly support emails and lots of new information to inspire
you. Come and join the Supercharge Your Gut Program online at
superchargedfood.com and connect with the Supercharged
Food community.

To purchase my Love Your Gut Powder or Golden Gut Blend,
go to: superchargedfood.com/shop

COACH WITH ME

If you need a bit of extra help with your wellness goals, I offer
health coaching sessions in person or via Skype. The sessions
involve guiding you to make food and lifestyle choices to bring
your life back into balance. I offer a step-by-step holistic personal
health program to enable you to reach your current and future
health goals. If you'd like a personal session, contact me via email
on admin@superchargedfood.com

SOCIALISE WITH ME

blog: superchargedfood.com/blog
share: superchargedfood.com

 like: facebook.com/superchargedfood

 follow: twitter.com/LeeSupercharged

 insta: instagram.com/leesupercharged

 link: linkedin.com/in/leesupercharged

 watch: youtube.com/leeholmes67

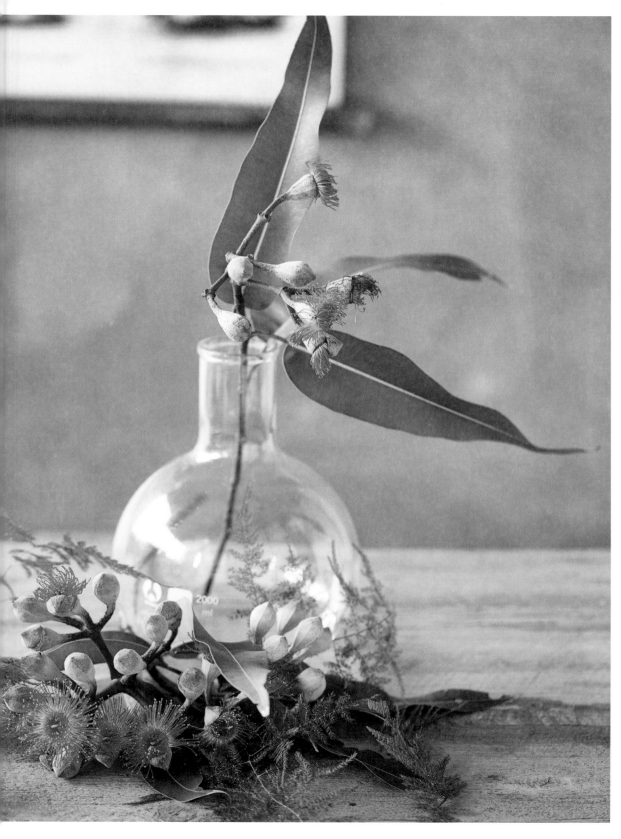

NOTES

For references to my website, see **superchargedfood.com**.
For references to my blog, see **superchargedfood.com/blog**.

1 (p. 17) Kobyliak N, *et al.* 'Probiotics in prevention and treatment of obesity: a critical view.' *Nutrition & Metabolism* 2016, vol. 13, no. 14; www.ncbi.nlm.nih.gov/pmc/articles/PMC4761174

2 (p. 18) Wong J, *et al.* 'Colonic health: fermentation and short chain fatty acids.' *Journal of Clinical Gastroenterology* 2006, vol. 40, no. 3, pp. 235–43; www.ncbi.nlm.nih.gov/pubmed/16633129

3 (p. 18) Den Besten G, *et al.* 'The role of short-chain fatty acids in the interplay between diet, gut microbiota, and host energy metabolism.' *Journal of Lipid Research* 2013, vol. 54, no. 9, pp. 2325–40; www.ncbi.nlm.nih.gov/pmc/articles/PMC3735932

4 (p. 18) Institute of Medicine (US) Food Forum. *The Human Microbiome, Diet, and Health: Workshop Summary.* Washington (DC): National Academies Press; 2013, 4, 'Influence of the microbiome on the metabolism of diet and dietary components'; www. ncbi.nlm.nih.gov/books/NBK154098

5 (p. 18) Mayo Clinic. 'Water: How much should you drink every day?'; www.mayoclinic.org/healthy-lifestyle/nutrition-and-healthy-eating/in-depth/water/art-20044256

6 (p. 20) Collins S and Bercik P. 'The relationship between intestinal microbiota and the central nervous system in normal gastrointestinal function and disease.' *Gastroenterology* 2009, vol. 136, no 6, pp. 2003–14; www.gastrojournal.org/article/S0016-5085(09)00346-1/fulltext

7 (p. 21) Zapata HJ and Quagliarello VJ. 'The microbiota and microbiome in aging: potential implications in health and age-related diseases.' *Journal of the American Geriatric Society* 2015, vol. 63, no. 4, pp. 776–81; www.ncbi.nlm.nih.gov/pmc/articles/PMC4406803

8 (p. 21) Lee Holmes, Supercharge Your Gut online summit; www.superchargedfood.com/blog/all/supercharge-your-gut-free-online-summit

9 (p. 29) Knowles SR, *et al.* 'Investigating the role of perceived stress on bacterial flora activity and salivary cortisol secretion: a possible mechanism underlying susceptibility to illness.' *Biological Psychology* 2008, no. 77, vol. 2, pp. 132–7; dx.doi.org/10.1016/j.biopsycho.2007.09.010

10 (p. 29) Foster JA and McVey Neufeld K. 'Gut brain axis: how the microbiome influences anxiety and depression.' *Trends in Neurosciences* 2013, vol. 36, no. 5, pp. 305–12; www.psych.ufl.edu/~dpdevine/bb/pelham.pdf

11 (p. 29) Bravo JA, *et al.* 'Ingestion of *Lactobacillus* strain regulates emotional behavior and central GABA receptor expression in a mouse via the vagus nerve.' *Proceedings of the National Academy of Sciences* 2011, vol. 108, no. 38, pp. 16050–55; www.ncbi.nlm.nih.gov/pmc/articles/PMC3179073

12 (p. 29) Hsiao, EY. 'The microbiota modulates gut physiology and behavioral abnormalities associated with autism.' *Cell* 2013, vol. 155, no. 7, pp. 1451–63; www.ncbi.nlm.nih.gov/pmc/articles/PMC3897394

13 (p. 30) EurekAlert, 12 April 2017. 'Gut microbes contribute to age-associated inflammation: Mouse study.' www.eurekalert.org/pub_releases/2017-04/cp-gmc040617.php

14 (p. 31) Goodrich JK, et al. 'Human genetics shape the gut microbiome.' Cell 2014, vol. 159, no. 4, pp. 789–99; www.ncbi.nlm.nih.gov/pmc/articles/PMC4255478

15 (p. 31) Diet vs Disease. 'Probiotics and weight loss review: microscopic miracle or mirage?'; www.dietvsdisease.org/probiotics-and-weight-loss-review

16 (p. 32) Osawa H. 'Ghrelin and Helicobacter pylori infection.' World Journal of Gastroenterology 2008, vol. 14, no. 41, pp. 6327–33; www.ncbi.nlm.nih.gov/pmc/articles/PMC2766113

17 (p. 34) Meissner HO, et al. 'Hormone-balancing effect of pre-gelatinized organic maca (Lepidium peruvianum Chacon): (I) Biochemical and pharmacodynamic study on maca using clinical laboratory model on ovariectomized rats.' International Journal of Biomedical Science 2006, vol. 2, no. 3, pp. 260–72; www.ncbi.nlm.nih.gov/pmc/articles/PMC3614604

18 (p. 37) Galland L. 'The gut microbiome and the brain.' Journal of Medicinal Food 2014, vol. 17, no. 12, pp. 1261–72; www.ncbi.nlm.nih.gov/pmc/articles/PMC4259177

19 (p. 38) National Institutes of Health. 'What makes you sleep?'; www.nhlbi.nih.gov/health/health-topics/topics/sdd/whatmakes

20 (p. 38) O'Mahony SM, et al. 'Serotonin, tryptophan metabolism and the brain-gut-microbiome axis.' Behavioural Brain Research 2015, vol. 277, pp. 32–48; www.sciencedirect.com/science/article/pii/S0166432814004768

21 (p. 47) Enck P, et al. 'Irritable bowel syndrome.' Nature Reviews Disease Primers 2016, vol. 2, article no. 16014; www.ncbi.nlm.nih.gov/pmc/articles/PMC5001845

22 (p. 53) Conlon MA and Bird AR. 'The impact of diet and lifestyle on gut microbiota and human health.' Nutrients 2015, vol. 7, no. 1, pp. 17–44; www.ncbi.nlm.nih.gov/pmc/articles/PMC4303825

23 (p. 54) Briani C, et al. 'Cobalamin deficiency: clinical picture and radiological findings.' Nutrients 2013; vol. 5, no. 11, pp 4521–39; www.ncbi.nlm.nih.gov/pmc/articles/PMC3847746

24 (p. 83) Saxena A, et al. 'Dietary agents and phytochemicals in the prevention and treatment of experimental ulcerative colitis.' Journal of Traditional and Complementary Medicine 2014, vol. 4, no. 4, pp. 203–17; www.ncbi.nlm.nih.gov/pmc/articles/PMC4220497

25 (p. 87) Konturek PC, et al. 'Stress and the gut: pathophysiology, clinical consequences, diagnostic approach and treatment options.' Journal of Physiological Pharmacology 2011, vol. 62, no. 6, pp. 591–99; www.jpp.krakow.pl/journal/archive/12_11/pdf/591_12_11_article.pdf

26 (p. 92) Forsythe P, et al. 'Vagal pathways for microbiome-brain-gut axis communication.' Advances in Experimental Medicine and Biology 2014, vol. 817, pp. 115–33; www.ncbi.nlm.nih.gov/pubmed/24997031

INDEX

ACKNOWLEDGEMENTS

My latest endeavour and exploration into the internal world of the gut hasn't been a solo effort — it's been a huge collaboration with people to whom I'd like to express my sincere thanks.

My publishers, Murdoch Books, and the ever beautiful Diana Hill, who has worked tirelessly on all of my books and who continues to be a huge source of support and encouragement. Diana is someone who allows me freedom of expression, but also knows how to draw the line at the odd buck crack joke. Thank you to Robert Gorman, Lou Johnson, Louise Cornege, Madeleine Kane, Sarah Odgers, Katie Bosher and Katri Hilden.

A very huge thank you to the stylish creative team: Grace Campbell, Steve Brown, Sarah O'Brien, makeup artist Emmily Banks and Coco Stallman, who all helped bring life and colour into this book. And to Luisa Brimble, for shooting the cover.

Special thanks to my friends, mentors and colleagues: my funny and hardworking assistant Toni Gam, researcher Shannon Young, contributors Dr Vincent Pedre, Yasmina Ykelenstam (Healing Histamine), Rebecca Coombes (The Healthy Gut), Fiona Tuck, Candice Kumai, Pia Larsen, Melissa Ambrosini, Rosana Lauria, Juliet Potter, Howard Porter, Georgie Bridge, Cindy Luken, Jessica Lowe, Lise Hearns, Kirsten Shanks, Vladia Cobradova and Marrianne Little.

Big love to my family Roxy, Arizona, Carol, Lorraine, Clive, Alex and Ben. My beautiful daughter and philosopher Tamsin Holmes, who will always be my closest friend, and Justin Andrew Smidmore my steadfast other half, whose support and love means everything to me.

Lee xo